HALSTEAD-REITAN
TEST BATTERY:
An Interpretive Guide

HALSTEAD-REITAN TEST BATTERY:
An Interpretive Guide

Paul E. Jarvis, Ph.D.
Fort Logan Mental Health Center
and
University of Denver
School of Professional Psychology
Denver, Colorado

Jeffrey T. Barth, Ph.D.
University of Virginia
School of Medicine
Charlottesville, Virginia

PAR Psychological Assessment Resources, Inc.
P.O. Box 998 / Odessa, Florida 33556 / Telephone (813) 968-3003

Jarvis, Paul E., 1931-
    Halstead-Reitan test battery.

    Bibliography: p.
    1. Halstead-Reitan Neuropsychological Test Battery.
2. Brain damage – Diagnosis. I. Barth, Jeffrey T.,
1949-   . II. Title.
RC386.6.H34J37 1984   616.8'0475   84-17809
ISBN 0-911907-01-7 (pbk.)

9 8 7 6 5 4   Printed in U.S.A.

Fourth Printing 1989

TABLE OF CONTENTS

Introduction

The purpose of this Guide is to teach a systematic method for addressing questions about brain damage that are frequently asked of clinicians. The data on which these answers are based are generated from the Halstead-Reitan Neuropsychological Test Battery. The proponents of this battery have repeatedly demonstrated a high degree of accuracy in answering these questions, but these accomplishments have often left neophyte neuropsychologist observers with more awe and admiration than understanding. A study of this Guide and the systematic application of the methods described herein should enable the reader to understand how these questions are answered and repeat the process with other cases.

Chapter 1 gives a brief rationale for the use of the Halstead-Reitan Battery. In Chapter 2 the tests of the battery are described, including the requirements for successful performance of them. The reader should note that the descriptions provided are not sufficient to enable one to administer the battery. Proper administration of the battery requires considerable training and practice and goes beyond the scope of this book. An understanding of the material in this chapter is, however, essential for adequate interpretation of the data.

Chapter 3 is the heart of the Guide. In it the methods of interpretation are described. New and esoteric techniques are not discussed, but a systematic approach to the data is provided. Compulsivity is the essence of this method. Swiercinsky (1978) has pointed out that accurate neuropsychological assessment depends not on how clever one is but on how thorough one is.

The next four chapters present a number of hypotheses regarding brain-behavior relationships pertinent to the data derived from the battery. There are no original research results presented here; instead, relationships which have previously been reported in the literature or presented in lecture form by recognized experts are described. Many of these have been demonstrated empirically, while some are part of the "neuropsychological folklore"; references are therefore provided only where there is a clear source. The relationships presented were chosen on the basis of their utility in both clinical work and in teaching this method of interpretation. As such, the reader is cautioned to regard them and use them as hypotheses and not as doctrines.

The reader will note that many of these hypotheses are repeated several times across chapters. This redundancy is intentional and serves two purposes. The first, for the reader who is relatively unfamiliar with the field, is a mnemonic one. Reading the same hypotheses over and over again will help fix them in memory and begin to clarify the relationships between factors such as test data, location of lesions, neuropathological processes, and so on. The second is a reference aid for the user of the Guide who is proceeding through the steps in the method of interpretation. This redundancy ensures that the relevant hypotheses will be encountered at each step as one proceeds through them.

Chapters 8, 9, and 10 take the reader beyond the specific methods for answering questions about brain damage solely from the data of the Battery. They provide information about other factors that need to be considered in "the real clinical world." Finally, Chapter 11 presents illustrations of the use of the method with clinical cases.

It is important to recognize that clinical neuropsychology is concerned with the study of brain-behavior relationships and the application of these principles to clinical problems. As such, *neurodiagnosis is not an end product,* nor for that matter, the most important aspect of a typical assessment. Rather, the evaluation and description of neuropathology is one step in an extensive process aimed at delineating a patient's cognitive and behavioral strengths and weaknesses, so that appropriate treatment and rehabilitation may be initiated. The determination of such intervention is based on many factors including severity, location and type of lesion, probable prognosis, intactness of cognitive and behavioral abilities, emotional stability, and social support systems. This guide focuses on the process involved in these necessary first steps of assessment, diagnosis, and description of the function of the brain, so that further decisions regarding implications for everyday functioning and eventual treatment may be made.

Chapter 1

THE SELECTION OF INSTRUMENTS
FOR
NEUROPSYCHOLOGICAL ASSESSMENT

SINGLE TESTS VS. BATTERIES OF TESTS

One of the first practical problems facing the psychologist who is unfamiliar with neuropsychological assessment is that of selecting the instrument or instruments to be used. For years psychologists have pursued the search for a quick, simple test for "organicity." This search has led from the Bender Visual Motor Gestalt Test (Bender, 1938) to other similar tests such as the Benton Visual Retention Test (Benton, 1963) and the Memory for Designs Test (Graham & Kendall, 1960), and continues with a proliferation of new, derivative forms of administration and scoring of the Bender such as the Background Interference Procedure (Canter, 1970). These references to a few of the best known single tests for brain damage only scratch the surface of the many procedures that have been considered, and in many instances, discarded with disillusionment over the years. In spite of this discouraging history, a new catalogue of psychological tests seldom passes over the practicing clinician's desk that does not include at least one offering of a "new, promising" instrument for the rapid assessment of brain damage.

Many of these instruments have been poorly evaluated and inadequately validated with appropriate experimental groups. Even those instruments which have been researched more carefully have usually shown little value in clinical practice for determining whether an individual patient has a cerebral lesion, and more importantly, what impact such neuropathology has on cognitive and behavioral abilities necessary for everyday functioning. The most common problem with regard to determining the presence or absence of a cerebral lesion with single tests has been the high number of false negative results

3

(Reitan, 1962). Russell (1975), for example, reported on a patient who had a severely damaged left cerebral hemisphere but was able to reproduce quite satisfactorily the designs on the Bender Visual Motor Gestalt Test. This type of performance is not at all uncommon. It is illustrated by the following case in which an 18-year-old male demonstrated a similarly retained ability in the presence of severe damage to the left cerebral hemisphere.

The drawings in Figure 1 were done two years after the patient had suffered a closed head injury in an automobile accident which left him blind in the left eye. Testing with the Halstead-Reitan Battery yielded an Impairment Index of .9 and considerable evidence that lateralized the damage to the left cerebral hemisphere, with the right hemisphere remaining relatively intact. The Bender Visual Motor Gestalt Test was not administered as part of the battery, but upon evaluation of the Halstead-Reitan Battery results, it was hypothesized that he should be able to perform adequately on visual-spatial tests such as the Benton Visual Retention Test and the Memory for Designs Test.

Evaluation of the patient's performance on the Benton Visual Retention Test suggested only that his performance "raises the question of impairment," and assessment of performance on the Memory for Designs Test did not indicate any neurological impairment, since he made only one scoreable error on all of the designs. It is also interesting to note that this patient was still able to play quite a good game of chess following this severe injury, relying heavily on his relatively intact right cerebral hemisphere to visualize the positions of pieces on the board and the sequences of moves.

Cases such as this illustrate the danger of using a single test for "organicity" since any such measure can tap only a few of the many aspects of behavior and cognition that are mediated by the cerebral hemispheres. Brain damage is not a unitary concept, but rather multidimensional, and cannot be evaluated utilizing a unidimensional model of assessment.

CHOICE OF A BATTERY

The problems of unidimensional models clearly argue for the use of a battery of tests which will assess performance in a number of different behavioral areas dependent upon the integration of different cerebral systems. A number of authors, including Lezak (1983) and Luria (1966, 1973) have advocated the use of test batteries that are individually tailored to assess the problems of patients on a case by case basis. Golden summarized the arguments for this approach when he stated that "it acknowledges the individuality of the patient's deficits and attempts to adapt the examination to this individuality" (Golden, 1978, p. 48). He also indicated that the examiner should concentrate on those problem areas that seem most important. According to this approach, for example, an examination of a patient who presented with primary problems in the language area might be given a thorough aphasia examination, while

FIGURE 1

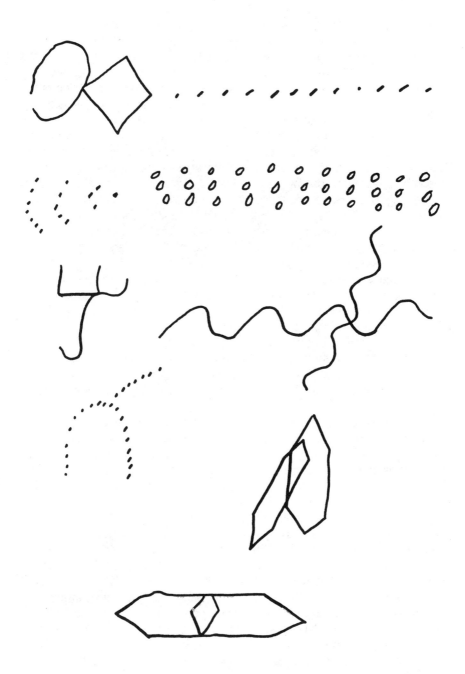

sensory and motor functions could be tested less thoroughly, if at all. This would represent major time and cost savings.

On the other hand, Halstead (1947) and Reitan (e.g., 1974), and more recently many of Reitan's students, have advocated the use of a standard battery of neuropsychological tests – specifically the Halstead-Reitan Battery. This battery (described in Chapter 2) is well-known and is by far the most thoroughly validated and standardized. The brain-behavior relationships which are important to the clinician in making diagnostic and prognostic statements and formulating rehabilitation plans have been more clearly and consistently demonstrated with this battery than with other existing batteries.

The Halstead-Reitan Battery taps most major functional areas that are of concern to the clinical neuropsychologist; therefore, unsuspected deficits are not missed as might be the case with a more focused approach. For example, a patient whose primary presenting symptoms were language difficulties might also have subtle sensory or motor deficits which would be revealed by this Battery. The use of the Halstead-Reitan Battery also allows for the application of the several different inferential approaches to interpretation of neuropsychological data suggested by Reitan (1967) and described in Chapter 3.

Another advantage of the use of this battery is that in many centers throughout the country there are data from a large number of cases in which neurological diagnosis has been validated by physical procedures, including neurosurgery and autopsy. Clinicians collecting this same "standard" data can check their hypotheses on individual cases under question with data from other cases in which the neurological diagnosis has been established. Similarly, the use of this battery also allows the clinician to contribute additional data to this pool of information for research purposes without additional effort and expense.

The use of a standard battery also allows the use of trained technicians to administer the test, saving the time of the neuropsychologist for interpretation and treatment planning. Some have argued that by using technicians the psychologist has limited contact with the patient, thereby reducing the opportunity to apply a high level of "clinical skill" in the assessment process. This objection can be addressed in the following way. The psychologist may routinely interview each patient either before or after the testing. It may be particularly valuable for the psychologist to interview the patient after the testing and after a preliminary review of the test results. This may be done using the interview outline suggested in Chapter 8. For example, if sensory or motor deficits are seen in the test results, the psychologist may question the patient about his or her awareness of them, their onset, and how they affect the patient's everyday functioning (many times people are not aware of deficits which are identified by these tests). This may also provide an opportunity for the psychologist to make initial suggestions for coping with some impairments. For example, a person who has only minimal awareness of a deficit in one sensory modality may receive some immediate benefit from attempts to rely more heavily on an intact modality to improve some aspect of daily functioning.

The use of the standard Halstead-Reitan Battery is recommended for all of the above reasons, but with certain modifications in order to increase the amount and value of the data obtained. The first step in this process is to attempt the standard administration of all tests in the battery. If the patient is unable to perform the tests under the standard procedures or performs poorly, the examiner should record observations about how and why the person appeared to fail to perform adequately under standard conditions. These may include factors such as peripheral sensory or motor damage, deficits in attention, or fatigue.

The next step is what Lezak (1983) has called "testing the limits." That is, if a person is making progress on a time limited test such as Block Design of the WAIS, the examiner should allow continuation beyond the limits until further progress cannot be made or until the item is completed. This yields two scores, a "standard" score and a "maximum possible" score, as well as an indication of how far below the norms the performance is with the standardized administration. If two patients have not completed all of the blocks on an item of the Block Design Test by the end of the time limit (e.g., 120 seconds), they would both obtain a zero for that item, and no difference in performance could be determined from that data alone. However, if both are allowed to continue beyond 120 seconds, and one completes the design successfully in 125 seconds, and the other completes it only after 240 seconds or fails to complete it at all, considerable additional information is available. This information has implications for the nature of the functional deficit as well as for rehabilitation planning. The patient who completes the design in 125 seconds may have been slowed by coordination problems or by psychomotor retardation which is part of a depressive syndrome, and this may have implications for psychotherapy. On the other hand, the person who never completes the design may be impaired by a deficit in ability to deal with spatial relationships, which would suggest structuring a rehabilitation plan which minimizes the need for this particular skill.

After standard administration procedures have been attempted, extensive behavioral observations regarding performance recorded, and, when appropriate, testing the limits has been accomplished, the examiner may wish to modify procedures for some tests to refine the judgments concerning the reasons for poor performance. For example, if performance on the Seashore Rhythm or Speech-sounds Perception Test is extremely poor as the apparent result of inability to sustain attention for the necessary time, the test or tests may be readministered at a slower pace to determine whether the patient can identify differences in rhythmic patterns or differences in phonemes when the requirement for sustained attention is changed.

The neuropsychologist may also decide to add additional tests to more fully explore deficits identified or suggested by tests in the standard battery.

For example, if a difficulty in copying the simple geometric designs on the Reitan-Indiana Aphasia Screening Test is observed, it may not be clear whether this results from a motor problem or a deficiency in processing spatial relationships. The former may be clarified by the administration of tests such as the Kløve-Matthews Motor Steadiness Battery (Reitan & Davison, 1974) and the latter by the administration of a test such as the Benton Visual Retention Test (Benton, 1963) or the Benton Judgment of Line Orientation Test (Benton, 1978).

Most neuropsychologists who have agreed with the advantages of using the standard Halstead-Reitan Test Battery have found that there are some functional areas which do not appear to be tapped adequately by this battery. They have, therefore, added other tests to their administration such as the Wechsler Intelligence Scales, which are not a standard part of the battery. Other useful additions include the Wechsler Memory Scale (1945) with the modification suggested by Russell (1975), and the Minnesota Multiphasic Personality Inventory. Some neuropsychologists prefer to include other tests of verbal and nonverbal memory, and the Kløve-Matthews Motor Steadiness Battery is also commonly included. In spite of Reitan's (1955) finding that Critical Flicker Frequency (CFF) does not contribute to the overall discrimination between brain-damaged and normal groups of subjects, a measure of CFF is a potentially useful addition to the battery. While a test of CFF is not useful in identifying brain damage in general, it can aid in identifying patients with multiple sclerosis (MS), which is a progressive neurological disorder that can be confused with a variety of other neurological and psychiatric conditions. Jarvis and Buchholz (1981) identified 70% of patients with MS without misidentifying any neurologically normal subjects. This procedure only adds about 15 minutes of testing time, but the equipment required is specialized and expensive (about $900), so it is not widely utilized. The only constraint here appears to be the practical one of the resources required. In many laboratories it is highly desirable to limit the amount of testing done to that which can be accomplished within a reasonable time period, which is often defined as 6-8 hours.

For all of these reasons, the use of the Halstead-Reitan Battery with the suggested modifications and possible additions is recommended. The method of interpretation presented in this Guide is based on this expanded and modified battery.

Chapter 2

DESCRIPTION
OF THE
HALSTEAD-REITAN
NEUROPSYCHOLOGICAL BATTERY

Halstead (1947) originally employed a battery of 27 measures in his study of cerebral functioning and biological intelligence. From these he eventually selected 10 measures which contributed to the Halstead Impairment Index. Reitan (1955) later discarded three of these measures which were based on the Time/Sense Test and the Critical Flicker Frequency procedure, since he found they did not contribute significantly to the discrimination of brain-damaged from intact patients. The Halstead-Reitan Neuropsychological Test Battery today consists of eight tests which will be described below. (The complete instructions for administration of these tests are given in Reitan's *Manual for Administration of Neuropsychological Test Batteries for Adults and Children,* undated.)

CATEGORY TEST

The first of these measures is the Category Test. For this test the patient is seated in front of an opaque glass screen on which 208 stimulus slides are serially projected. Located below the screen are the response keys, which consist of four numbered lights with a spring-loaded switch below each light. The patient is told that he/she will see a series of slides on the screen and that each slide will remind the patient of a number between 1 and 4. The patient is instructed to push the switch corresponding to the number that he/she is reminded of and that a correct response will result in a positive reinforcement (a bell). On the other hand, when the patient presses the switch corresponding to an incorrect answer, he/she receives a negative reinforcement (a noxious-sounding buzzer). The test is divided into seven subtests and the patient is told that there is a common principle or idea that governs the determination of the correct response in each subtest. The first subtest has a very simple principle: The patient is required only to match the Roman Numeral which appears on the screen with the Arabic Numeral on the response unit. In the second subtest, the patient is required to give a response corresponding to the number of items (circles, squares, etc.) appearing on the screen. As the subtests progress, the stimuli and the principles determining the correct answers become more complex. For example, stimuli may differ along several dimensions such as size, shape, color, position, and density of the figure. (See Reitan & Davison, 1974, for a more complete description of the stimuli in the more complex subtests.) The seventh and final subtest is different in that the correct answer is not determined by any single principle; instead, this subtest repeats items from the first six subtests. Therefore, it introduces a memory component, rather than requiring new concept information.

This test is a complex test of new problem solving, judgment, abstract reasoning, concept formation, mental flexibility, and mental efficiency. It requires a number of "higher order" functions such as the ability to note similarities and differences in the stimuli and to formulate hypotheses regarding the principle that determines the correct answer. It is also a test of learning ability utilizing nonverbal material. Finally, there is a memory component to the test that not only requires the patient to remember which principle was correct in determining the answer to an individual problem item, but also in subtest 7, requires a longer recall of previously learned correct reponses.

The examiner's role in the administration of this test, as in all of the other tests of the battery, is to give precisely the same standardized instructions to each patient. Furthermore, the examiner needs to make every effort to elicit the best possible performance on the part of the patient. Various types of assistance may be given in doing this, including prompting, elaboration, or repetition of various points in the instructions. Verbal positive or negative reinforcement may be given in addition to the bell or buzzer for correct or incorrect responses. The examiner must never, however, give the patient the principle(s) involved in any of the subtests. The total number of errors is the score which contributes to the Halstead Impairment Index.

There are relatively few pitfalls in the administration of the Category Test; however, some patients will attempt to make a second response when the first response to a stimulus is incorrect. Patients should be told that this is not allowed and if the patient shows a tendency toward this behavior, the examiner should anticipate this and make every effort to prevent the patient from making a second response following an incorrect one.

Subtest 3 is radically different from and more difficult than the first two subtests and, for that reason, must be treated differently. It is important to encourage the patient to concentrate on the task at hand, particularly during the first several slides of this subtest, to ensure the best possible performance and to limit discouragement and resignation to failure.

Although the Category Test is not timed, it is common practice to limit response time for each item to 15-20 seconds.

TACTUAL PERFORMANCE TEST

The Tactual Performance Test (TPT) is a test which utilizes an apparatus similar to the Seguin-Goddard Formboard. In the administration of this test, the patient is blindfolded and seated in front of a form board on a supporting rack. The patient is never allowed to see the board or the blocks. The 10 blocks which fit on the board are placed on the table immediately in front of the patient and below the board. The examiner quickly runs the patient's hand over the board and blocks to familiarize him/her with the nature of the task. The patient is then told to place the blocks which are in front of him/her in the correct slots on the board. This is a timed test and the patient is encouraged to perform the task as quickly as possible. The patient first performs the task with only the dominant hand. When this is completed, the blindfold is kept on and the blocks are removed from the board and replaced in front of the patient. The patient then performs this same task with the nondominant hand. The blindfold is kept on, the blocks are once again removed from the board, and the patient then performs the task with both hands. The three trials are timed with a maximum of 10 minutes per trial unless the patient is close to completion at the 10 minute mark with the dominant hand. In that case, each trial would be allowed to continue for a maximum of 15 minutes. Next, while the blindfold is kept on, the blocks and form board are removed and placed out of sight or covered up. The blindfold is then removed and the patient is given an 8½ × 11 sheet of white paper and a pencil and instructed to draw the outline of the form board with the blocks in the correct positions as nearly as he/she can remember them. Times and number of blocks placed correctly are recorded for the dominant hand, nondominant hand, and both hands. A total time is calculated and the number of blocks remembered and correctly located are recorded. This results, then, in a total of six scores – one each for the dominant hand, nondominant hand, both hands, total time, memory, and localization. These latter three – total time, memory, and localization – contribute to the Halstead Impairment Index.

In this complex test, the most obvious requirement for successful performance is the ability to sustain adequate strength and speed of movement. It also requires tactile perception and the ability to form a visual "map" of the board. Since the patient is not told until after the third trial that he/she will be required to draw the board, there is an additional requirement for incidental memory.

There are a number of potential problems in the administration of this test. The first of these involves the adequacy of the blindfold. Since the test is completely useless if the patient ever sees the blocks or the board, this is a crucial requirement. The adequacy of the blindfold can be checked by making a "threatening" movement of the examiner's hand towards the patient's eyes from below to see whether the patient can see this. It may be necessary to repeat this at times during the test. Since many patients find the blindfold uncomfortable, either physically or psychologically, they have a tendency to take it off as soon as they think the test is done. Consequently, it is important for the examiner to say "keep the blindfold on" at the end of each trial and to make certain that it is kept in place after the third trial until the form board and blocks are all out of sight.

Many patients will also have a tendency to use both hands on either one or both of the trials which they are required to perform with one hand only. Similarly, they sometimes have a tendency to shift to the dominant hand when the nondominant hand is being tested. The examiner should be aware of these natural tendencies and stop the patient quickly if he/she attempts to do so. It is often helpful to have the patient sit close to the edge of the table with the hand that is not being examined on his/her knee beneath the surface of the table, or even under their own knee. This makes it more difficult for the patient to shift hands inadvertently, as the hand that is not being examined will be stopped by the table if there is a tendency to utilize it.

SEASHORE RHYTHM TEST

The Seashore Rhythm Test was adapted from the Seashore Tests of Musical Ability. This test is administered by playing a tape recording which represents 30 pairs of rhythmic beats. The patient's task is to record on an answer sheet an "S" or a "D" indicating whether the second group of beeps in each pair was the same as, or different from, the first group of beeps in the pair. For example, the patient may hear a pair of beats that sounds like this:

beep—beep beep beep—beep
beep—beep beep beep—beep

The correct response to this stimulus is "S or Same." Alternatively the subject may hear a pair like this:

beep beep—beep beep beep—beep
beep beep—beep beep—beep beep

The correct response to this stimulus is "D or Different." The pace of this recording is quite rapid and no cues are given as to the number of the stimulus pair or the corresponding number on the answer sheet for the 10 pairs of beeps within any of the 3 subtests. The number of correct responses (or rank score) contributes to the Impairment Index.

The most obvious requirement for the successful performance of this test is the ability to discriminate between different patterns of nonverbal sounds.

In addition, however, this test requires the ability to sustain attention and concentration without any cues as to where one should be on the response sheet. A significant degree of coordination among ear, eye, and hand is also necessary. A poor performance on this test, then, may have little to do with inability to discriminate auditory rhythmic patterns, but may indicate a severe impairment of attention, concentration or coordination.

SPEECH-SOUNDS PERCEPTION TEST

The Speech-sounds Perception Test is also administered with a tape recorder. On this test the patient has a response sheet with 60 groups of 4 "nonsense words," which all contain the "ee" sound. The patient's task is to listen to the tape and underline the correct nonsense word. For example, the first stimulus word is "theets" and the patient must choose the correct response on the answer sheet from the words, "theeks, zeeks, theets, and zeets." The patient then hears "the second word is weej." The patient's task is to underline the correct word from among "weech, yeech, weej, and yeej." While this test is longer in duration than the Seashore Rhythm Test, having 60 stimuli as opposed to 30, the pace is much slower and the patient is cued prior to each stimulus regarding where on the answer sheet a response should be marked. The number of errors on this test contributes to the Impairment Index.

The most obvious way in which the Speech-sounds Perception Test differs from the Seashore Rhythm Test is that the stimuli are verbal ones as opposed to nonverbal rhythms. In addition, the pace is slower and the patient is given cues about where the responses should be marked on the answer sheet. The requirement for attention and concentration is more sustained, yet the task is somewhat simpler than that of the Rhythm Test since more cues are provided. The same requirements for ear, eye, hand coordination, and the same possibilities for interference with adequate performance are present on both tests.

FINGER OSCILLATION TEST

The Finger Oscillation or Finger Tapping Test requires that the patient tap as rapidly as possible with the index finger on a small lever which is attached to a mechanical counter. The patient is given five consecutive 10-second trials with the preferred hand and then five consecutive trials with the nonpreferred hand. The scores on this test are the average number of taps in a 10-second period for the dominant hand and a 10-second period for the nondominant hand. The score on the dominant hand contributes to the Halstead Impairment Index. This test is basically a test of simple motor speed, although some degree of coordination is required.

It is important in the administration of this test for the examiner to start the stopwatch or clock at the precise moment the patient taps the lever the first time. Similarly, it is important to note whether the patient continues to tap after the examiner says "stop" and if so, to subtract the number of extra taps from the score. It is also important to make sure that the patient is using only the index finger in tapping and is not making extraneous movements of the entire hand or arm. This can generally be assured by making certain that the heel of the patient's hand remains flat on the table. Some patients will show a great deal of intertrial variability in speed, and it is important to get *five consecutive* trials which are within five taps of each other in terms of speed. It may be difficult to achieve this with some patients, and one may need to administer as many as 10 trials in cases of extreme variability. No more than 10 trials should be administered, and one may then drop the fastest and the slowest trials and take an average of the remaining eight trials as the score for that hand. Even though this test was developed and validated with the above instructions, many laboratories have begun to utilize an alternative method of administration to eliminate some of the between trial variability and fatigue by alternating trials between the dominant and nondominant hands. This appears acceptable if interpretation of absolute value is of secondary importance to the issue of right/left differences and traditional norms are not being used.

HALSTEAD IMPAIRMENT INDEX

The Halstead Impairment Index is computed from the seven scores derived from the above tests. The computation of this index is described in the section on scoring of the individual tests.

TRAIL MAKING TEST

Even though the Trail Making Test does not contribute to the Halstead Impairment Index, it is considered an integral part of the Halstead-Reitan Battery. The Trail Making Test is a timed paper and pencil test which consists of Parts A and B. On each part the patient is given a sample page which is used for practice to aid the patient in understanding the instructions. The examiner then gives the patient Part A, which is a white sheet of paper with 24 numbered circles distributed in a random pattern. The patient is required to connect the circles with lines in numerical order as quickly as possible. Part B, which is given after practice on a sample sheet, consists of 25 circles – some of which are numbered from 1 to 13 and the remainder lettered from A to L. The patient is required to connect the circles beginning with number 1, then going to A, and from A to 2, 2 to B, and so on, in an alternating sequence. The scores on this test are the total times in seconds for each part and the number of errors.

Part A requires that the patient be able to scan the page rapidly, finding the correct numbers and connecting them in numerical sequence. In addition to the perceptual and problem solving requirements, it includes a significant requirement for motor speed and coordination. Part B has the same requirements but, in addition, the patient must be able to recognize the different significance of the two types of symbols within the circles, and to alternate from one set of symbols to the other appropriately and consistently. The patient must simultaneously maintain attention on two aspects of a stimulus situation.

The most common problem in the administration of this test is that of quickly correcting the patient's errors. If the patient makes an error, the clock is kept running and the examiner must rapidly and efficiently indicate that the move was an error and return the patient to the last correct point in the sequence with the instruction to continue. This requires that the examiner be constantly alert to the patient's performance and thoroughly familiar with the positions of the numbered and lettered circles on the page so that he/she can correct patient errors without unduly penalizing the patient in terms of the timed score.

APHASIA SCREENING TEST

Most examiners using this battery follow Reitan's example by incorporating the Aphasia Screening Test, which was prepared by Reitan as a modification of the Halstead-Wepman Aphasia Screening Test. The stimuli for this test are incorporated into a small spiral bound notebook. The first stimulus is a picture of a square which the patient is asked to draw on a sheet of paper without lifting the pencil from the paper. This procedure is often repeated to see if the drawing improves on a second trial. The patient is then asked to name the object and then to spell it.

The second and third stimuli are drawings of a Greek cross and a triangle. The patient is asked in sequence once again to draw them (twice), name them, and spell them. This is followed by a drawing of a baby which the patient is asked to name.

The next stimulus is a picture of a clock. The patient is asked not to say anything about it, but just to write the name of the picture on the paper. A drawing of a fork is next and the patient is asked to name it.

The patient is asked to read out loud the next four stimulus cards which have the following on them:

"7 six 2"

"MGW"

"See the black dog"

"He is a friendly animal, a famous winner of dog shows"

The following three items are presented verbally, and the patient is asked to repeat them after the examiner. These items are "triangle," "Massachu-setts," and "Methodist Episcopal." Next the patient is shown a card with the word "SQUARE" and asked not to say the word but to write it on the paper. Then the patient is shown a card with the word "SEVEN" on it and asked to read it out loud. Then he/she is asked to repeat the word "seven" after the examiner. Next, the patient is asked to repeat, "He shouted the warning" after the examiner and then to explain the meaning of that sentence. The patient is then asked to write the sentence on the paper.

The patient is then requested to write down the problem "85 – 27" on a piece of paper and to perform the calculation. The next item is also an arithmetic problem, "17 × 3," which the patient is asked to do mentally and to write down only the answer. The patient is then shown a picture of a key and asked to name it. The examiner then says, "If you had one of these in your hand, show me how you would use it." Then the patient is asked to copy the picture of the key on paper.

A card is then shown to the patient which reads, "Place left hand to right ear." The examiner asks the patient to read the card and then to do what it says on the card. Finally, the examiner says "Now I want you to put your left hand to your left elbow."

It is obvious that the Aphasia Screening Test taps a number of different areas of dysfunction. These include dysnomia, dyslexia, spelling dyspraxia, dyscalculia, and constructional dyspraxia. Patients may make a variety of errors on this test for many reasons that having nothing to do with brain dysfunction, and it is obvious that educational deficits can affect abilities such as reading, spelling, and calculation. Similarly, psychiatric disturbances which include thought disorder may result in a variety of errors. The most important consideration for the examiner is that all responses must be recorded verbatim, with the exception of absolutely correct responses which are given without any hesitation or delay. Only in this way is it possible to interpret these responses and their relationship to etiologic factors.

SENSORY PERCEPTUAL EXAMINATION

The addition of the Reitan-Kløve Sensory Perceptual Examination to the battery augments the assessment of "higher order" functions by including procedures which are common to most clinical neurological examinations. Administration of these procedures in a reliable manner requires a good deal of skill and practice by the examiner. They can only be learned by practicing under the guidance of an experienced examiner; therefore, only a brief description of these procedures will be given here. Tactile, auditory, and visual modalities are tested to make certain that the patient can perceive a very low intensity stimulus delivered unilaterally. Stimuli are then delivered bilaterally and simultaneously. Tactile stimuli are very light touches presented to the hands and face while the patient's eyes are closed. Auditory stimuli are presented from behind the patient by the examiner's rubbing the thumb and finger together gently next to the patient's ear. In the testing of visual perception the examiner sits in front of the patient and makes a slight movement of the fingers at the periphery of the patient's vision while the patient focuses on the bridge of the examiner's nose. Visual fields are checked by a gross direct confrontation method.

Further tests of tactile perception include a test of tactile finger recognition in which the patient is asked, with eyes closed, to identify the individual fingers that are touched by the examiner on each hand. In the fingertip number writing test, the patient is asked to identify numbers written with a stylus on the fingertips of his/her hand by the examiner while the patient's eyes are closed. Finally, the tactile coin recognition task requires the patient to identify through touch alone pennies, nickels, and dimes.

The Reitan-Kløve Tactile Form Recognition Test was developed separately from the rest of the Sensory Perceptual Examination, but is usually recorded on the same form. This procedure requires the patient to identify flat plastic shapes (cross, square, triangle, and circle) which are placed in the patient's hand after being inserted through a curtained opening in a vertical board. On the side of the board facing the patient is another set of the same stimulus figures (cross, square, triangle, and circle). The patient is instructed to point to the same figure which is being presented in the hand hidden by the board.

It is obvious that these procedures require adequate functioning in the tactile, auditory, and visual modalities. A comparison of the number of errors on the two sides of the body is, then, the critical data obtained from this portion of the battery. One of the most important kinds of information obtained is that concerning suppressions, or the failure to perceive a sensation on one side of the body when both sides are simultaneously stimulated.

The importance and significance of data about suppressions makes it imperative that the examiner determine initially that the patient is able to perceive unilateral stimulation. Sometimes in the auditory modality, for example, a patient will have a higher threshold for perception on one side of the body than on the other. This may require the examiner to present simultaneous stimulation of unequal intensity in order to eliminate different threshold levels and purely test for cortical suppression. Another problem that many patients have is focusing steadily on the bridge of the examiner's nose during the visual portions of the examination. The examiner must be aware of any eye movement on the part of the patient and repeat instructions and procedures if necessary. It is also important to remember that this is essentially a physical examination – an assessment of tactile, auditory, and verbal perception – and is not an assessment of verbalization, memory, or attention. On the fingertip number writing test, for example, it is common to find patients who give responses other than the numbers included in the instructions and demonstration (3, 4, 5, 6). When numbers such as 2, 7, or 8 are given as responses, it is clear that the patient either has not understood or retained the instructions, or is not paying attention to the task. In this case, instructions may be repeated or "X"s and "O"s substituted for the numbers to be drawn on the fingertips.

STRENGTH OF GRIP

A measure of Strength of Grip obtained with the Smedley hand dynamometer has also routinely been added to the battery by Reitan and others. This test is very simple and requires only a few minutes to administer. The instrument is adjusted to accommodate the size of the patient's hand, and the patient is instructed to stand, holding the instrument at his/her side, pointed toward the floor with the arm held straight at the elbow. The patient is simply instructed to squeeze the dynamometer as hard as he/she can. Alternating trials are given with the dominant and nondominant hands with a total of two trials for each hand.

This is a simple measure of motor strength with no other behavioral components required for adequate performance. There do not appear to be any common problems in administering the test. Unlike the Finger Oscillation Test, it is quite easy to get fairly consistent measures on repeated trials, and a large number of trials is rarely required.

WECHSLER SCALES AND MINNESOTA
MULTIPHASIC PERSONALITY INVENTORY

Either the Wechsler Bellevue Intelligence Test or the Wechsler Adult Intelligence Scale have routinely been administered as part of the standard neuropsychological test battery. The Minnesota Multiphasic Personality Inventory is often administered in order to give additional information about the psychological functioning of patients. Since these tests should be well known to the readers of this Guide, no further comments will be offered.

SCORING, CUT-OFF SCORES, AND DATA SHEETS

Scoring

Scoring of tests on the battery ranges from simple, objective, and almost automatic procedures on some tests to complex, relatively subjective, and more time-consuming methods on others. The scoring of the Category Test is an example of the former, since the score is simply the total number of errors made by the patient in responding to the 208 stimulus slides. On this test, there is no ambiguity about the scoring since an error is indicated to the examiner by the sound of the buzzer. If, as unfortunately sometimes happens, the patient immediately corrects his/her response and gives a correct response, this is scored as an error, and every attempt is made to prevent the patient from giving more than one response to future items.

There are six scores that are recorded for the TPT. For the dominant hand, the time required to place all 10 blocks correctly is recorded. If the patient has not placed all 10 blocks correctly within 10 minutes, the time is recorded as 10 minutes and the number of blocks placed in 10 minutes is recorded in parentheses. The same procedure is followed for the nondominant hand, and for both hands. If on the first trial the patient has nearly all of the blocks in at the end of 10 minutes, the examiner may permit the patient to continue working but should record the number of blocks placed after 10 minutes as well as the total time required to place all 10 blocks correctly. The total time is simply a sum of the time on the first three trials. The examiner should also indicate the number of blocks correctly placed for the total of the three trials. If the patient continued to work for more than 10 minutes on the first trial, the examiner should allow the patient the same amount of time on subsequent trials to provide consistency and aid in proper interpretation of right/left differences.

Obtaining the memory score for the TPT is more difficult and somewhat subjective. The important thing to remember is that scoring for memory is very liberal. If a patient either draws a block correctly or names a drawing correctly, even though the drawing does not resemble the named block, credit is given for that drawing. This measure is not a test of verbal ability or drawing skill, but simply a measure of incidental memory. When the patient has completed the drawing of the board with whatever encouragement is needed (without specific hints) to remember any missing pieces, the examiner should question the patient about the name of any ambiguously drawn block. Even if a drawing is not recognizable as any one of the blocks and if the patient gives it a name which corresponds (at least approximately) to the name of the shape of a block, credit is given for that figure.

Scoring of the localization component is also quite difficult at times. The easiest way to score for localization is to divide the outline of the board which the patient used and to position the blocks into nine sectors as indicated in Figure 2. The examiner should then give localization credit for any block whose major portion falls within the proper sector of the drawing in relationship to similar sectors on the board itself.

Three of these six scores – total time, memory, and localization – are included in the Halstead Impairment Index. The other three scores – the times for dominant hand, nondominant hand, and both hands – are not included in the Impairment Index. They are examined using a different method of inference and have strong implications for lateralization of cerebral dysfunction.

The score on the Finger Oscillation Test is an objective one that is relatively easily obtained, although there may be difficulties during the administration of the test in obtaining consistency of performance for the required number of trials. The scores that are recorded are the average number of taps in 10 seconds with the dominant hand and the average number of taps in 10 seconds with the nondominant hand. The score with the dominant hand enters into the Halstead Impairment Index. As was indicated above for the TPT, the comparison of the scores on the dominant and nondominant hand is considered from the perspective of a different method of inference and has strong implications for lateralization of cerebral dysfunction.

FIGURE 2

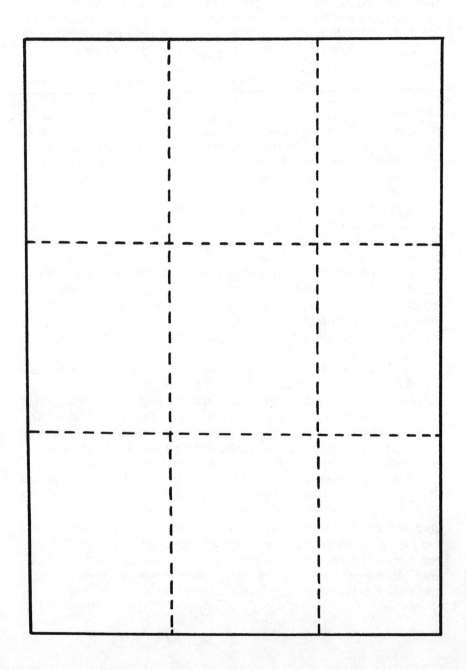

Cut-Off Scores For Brain Damage

The cut-off scores which best separate groups of brain-damaged from non-brain-damaged subjects as reported by Reitan (1959) are shown in Table 1. The value of the Impairment Index obviously decreases as the number of test scores available declines and it is of little value when the number of scores available is less than five (see Table 3 for calculation of Impairment Index based upon 7, 6, or 5 tests).

The other tests which are commonly included in a standard battery do not have cut-off scores, and in some cases do not really lend themselves to calculating numerical scores. Instead, they are more often either evaluated from the perspective of the difference in performance on the two sides of the body or examined for evidence of pathognomonic signs. Strength of Grip is a measure which tends to fall into the former category. While one expects most adult female patients to have a strength of grip of at least 20 kilograms in the dominant hand and most adult male patients to have a strength of grip of at least 40 kilograms with the dominant hand, the more important consideration by far is the relationship of the two hands. One generally expects to find that the dominant hand will be 10% greater than the strength of the nondominant hand. Deviations from this expectation may have implications for lateralization of cerebral impairment.

The Aphasia Screening Test is an example where pathognomonic signs may be the most useful data. While Russell, Neuringer, and Goldstein (1970) have developed a scoring system for the Aphasia Screening Test specifically for research purposes, quality of response is exceedingly important and may not lend itself to quantitative scoring. Certain types of clearly dysphasic errors must be considered to be pathognomonic signs, and one or two of them would clearly have more significance in terms of interpretation than a greater number of more equivocal errors. This is further complicated by the fact that interpretation of responses to the Aphasia Screening Test must take into consideration such factors as intelligence and education.

While interpretation of the Sensory Perceptual Examination is based more on inferences regarding differences in performance of the two sides of the body, there are also some pathognomonic signs which may be seen. Consistent, reliable suppressions on one side of the body in a single sensory modality should be considered to be a pathognomonic sign since such suppressions are seldom found among intact patients.

Since administration of a standard battery such as this generates a large amount of raw data, it is helpful to use a form for recording a summary of the results. There is probably no special virtue in any single form and the major value of any summary form is to provide a consistent format for the organization and evaluation of results. Figure 3 offers an example of a summary data sheet which combines many of the positive aspects of several forms.

TABLE 1

Halstead Cut-Off Scores Suggesting Brain Damage*

Tests	Halstead Cut-Off Scores
Category Test	51 or more errors
TPT Total Time	15.7 minutes or more
Memory	5 or less correct
Localization	4 or less correct
Seashore Rhythm	25 or less correct (6 or more rank score)
Speech-sounds Perception	8 or more errors
Finger Oscillation (Tapping) (Dominant hand)	50 or less taps in 10 seconds
Impairment Index	.5 or above

Normal	Mild	Moderate	Severe
0.0-0.2	0.3-0.4	0.5-0.7	0.8-1.0

The following test, while not contributing to the Halstead Impairment Index, has an established cut-off score for brain damage.

Trail Making	
Part A	40 seconds or more
Part B	91 seconds or more

*(From Reitan, 1955; 1959)

To calculate the Halstead Impairment Index, one divides the number of scores from Table 1 which are in the impaired range by the total number of tests given which contribute to the Halstead Impairment Index (maximum 7). This results in a decimal value between 0 and 1.0. If none of the scores were in the impaired range, the Impairment Index would be 0.0, while if all of them were in the impaired range (7 divided by 7, or 6 divided by 6, etc.), the Impairment Index would be 1.0. Since it is traditional to round off the results of this to the nearest 1 decimal place, the number of tests in the impaired range and the resulting impairment indices are listed on the prorated schedule on Table 3.

TABLE 2

Conversion Tables on Tests of the Halstead-Reitan Battery*

TPT Conversion of Seconds to Decimals		Seashore Rhythm Test Conversion of Raw Scores to Rank Scores	
		#Correct	Rank
1 - 3	0.0		
4 - 8	0.1		
9 - 15	0.2	29-30	1
16 - 20	0.3	28	2
21 - 27	0.4	27	3
28 - 32	0.5	26	5
33 - 39	0.6	25	6
40 - 44	0.7	24	8
45 - 51	0.8	23	9
52 - 56	0.9	22 & below	10
57 - 60	1.0		

*(From Reitan, 1955; 1959)

TABLE 3

Calculation of the Halstead Impairment Index Based on Number of Tests Used and Number of Test Scores which Fall Within the Brain-Impaired Range

Number of Halstead Tests Utilized

Number of Tests in Impaired Range

7 Tests	6 Tests	5 Tests
1 = 0.1	1 = 0.2	1 = 0.2
2 = 0.3	2 = 0.3	2 = 0.4
3 = 0.4	3 = 0.5	3 = 0.6
4 = 0.6	4 = 0.7	4 = 0.8
5 = 0.7	5 = 0.8	5 = 1.0
6 = 0.9	6 = 1.0	
7 = 1.0		

FIGURE 3

DATA SHEET
RESULTS OF NEUROPSYCHOLOGICAL EXAMINATION

Case Number:_____ Age:_____ Sex:_____ Education:_____ Handedness:_____

Name:_____ Employment:_____ IMPAIRMENT INDEX:_____ *

WAIS (or WAIS-R)

VIQ

PIQ

FS IQ

Scaled Scores

Information

Comprehension

Digit Span

Arithmetic

Similarities

Vocabulary

Picture Arrangement

Picture Completion

Block Design

Object Assembly

Digit Symbol

MINNESOTA MULTIPHASIC PERSONALITY
INVENTORY
(T-Scores)

?

L

F

K

Hs

D

Hy

Pd

Mf

Pa

Pt

Sc

Ma

Si

CATEGORY TEST   *

TACTUAL PERFORMANCE TEST

Time ——— # of Blks. In

Dominant hand:

Nondomin. hand:

Both hands:

Total Time: *

Memory: *

Localization: *

TRAIL MAKING TEST

Part A: [   ] seconds [   ] errors

Part B: [   ] seconds [   ] errors

SEASHORE RHYTHM TEST (correct)

Raw Score: [   ]   Rank: [   ] *

SPEECH-SOUNDS PERCEPTION TEST

Errors: *

FINGER OSCILLATION TEST

Dominant hand: *
Nondominant hand:

STRENGTH OF GRIP

Dominant hand: kilograms
Nondominant hand: kilograms

REITAN-KLØVE TACTILE FORM RECOGNITION TEST

Errors   Seconds

Dominant hand:

Nondominant hand:

SENSORY SUPPRESSIONS

Dominant:

Nondominant:

APHASIA SIGNS:

The scores which enter into the Halstead Impairment Index have asterisks on the far right hand side of the page so that it is easy to calculate the Impairment Index from those seven scores. The Impairment Index, the score on the Category Test, the localization score on the TPT, and the score on Part B of the Trail Making Test are those scores which are the most sensitive to brain damage; because these scores are generally examined first, they appear near the top of the list even though the Trail Making Test does not itself contribute to the Halstead Impairment Index.

Chapter 3

USE OF THE GUIDE

The following chapters contain a number of hypotheses regarding the brain-behavior relationships demonstrated by the data obtained from the Halstead-Reitan Battery. This selection of hypotheses is by no means all-inclusive of those that have appeared in the neuropsychological research literature; rather, those that appear in these chapters were selected on the basis of their clinical utility in neuropsychological assessment. Many of these hypotheses have become common knowledge in the field and may not be associated with specific research or references. No attempt has been made to indicate the nature or extent of validational studies regarding the selected hypotheses, and readers interested in pursuing this subject are urged to study the original research literature. Reitan (1975), for example, gives a review of a number of important validation studies and Hevern (1980) has reviewed more recent ones.

In performing a neuropsychological evaluation a number of questions should be answered. While there may at times be some variations, in general it is best to answer these questions in the sequence listed below:

1. **Is there cerebral impairment?** In asking this question we are essentially determining whether there is evidence of behavioral deficits (in the case of congenital damage), or behavioral changes (in the case of acquired lesions) that can be attributed to the presence of a brain lesion.

2. **What is the severity of the damage?** Here two questions are implied. The first is whether the severity of the damage is such that it is medically significant and requires medical and/or surgical intervention. The second is whether the severity of the damage is such that it will impair the person's ability to function in his/her daily activities.

27

3. Is the lesion progressive or static? This is obviously a matter of degree since there are some very slowly progressive, degenerative disorders and there are some very rapidly progressive, space occupying lesions, such as certain highly malignant neoplasms. The answer to this question has implications for whether a lesion is medically significant, as well as for prognosis.

4. Is the lesion diffuse, lateralized, or are there multiple lesions? Is the entire brain impaired, is one cerebral hemisphere primarily involved, or is there a "spotty" impairment with pockets of damage along with relatively unimpaired areas of the brain? Similarly, are all areas of functioning impaired to the same extent or are there more isolated areas of impairment of functioning with concomitant sparing?

5. Is the impairment in the anterior or posterior portions of the cerebral hemispheres and can it be localized? This is essentially a further refinement of question 4.

6. What is the most likely pathological process and what is the prognosis? It is often helpful in answering this question to first ask whether, on the basis of the answers to prior questions, certain pathological processes can be ruled out. For example, if the answer to question 3 is that the lesion is a static one, then one can rule out certain major categories of pathology such as rapidly growing neoplasms.

7. What are the individual's cognitive/behavioral strengths and weaknesses and how do they relate to daily living skills, treatment, and rehabilitation? *Even though this book focuses on the process of identifying brain-behavior relationships, the earlier questions (1-6) are ultimately aimed at answering this critical seventh question.*

It is important to answer certain questions in the above sequence. One cannot ascertain which hemisphere is most impaired if one has not first answered the question about whether a lesion is lateralized or not. Similarly, one cannot answer the question about the nature of the pathological process without having answered questions about severity, velocity, and location. It is not critical that certain questions be answered in precisely the order listed above. One can, for example, decide whether a lesion is more likely to be diffuse or lateralized before deciding on the probable velocity of the lesion. In general, however, it is helpful to address these questions in the sequence indicated above.

METHODS OF INFERENCE

This chapter will describe the use of the hypotheses presented in the following chapters in answering these seven questions. This approach is a multifaceted one which uses the four methods of inference suggested by Reitan (e.g., 1967). These are: 1) **level of performance,** 2) **patterns of scores on different tests and subtests,** 3) **differences in functioning of the different sides of the body,** and 4) **presence of pathognomonic signs.**

1) Assessment of **level of performance** is the most commonly used method of drawing inferences from test data. Most psychologists are familiar with this method of inference, having used it in evaluating data from intelligence tests and other types of assessment material. There is a long history, for example, in the psychological literature on tests such as the Benton Visual Retention Test (Benton, 1963), the Background Interference Procedures of Canter (1970), and the Memory for Designs Test (Graham & Kendall, 1960) which correlate the patient's overall level of performance with the presence or absence of brain damage. Chapter 1 presented the problems inherent in the use of any single test for making inferences about this question. The sole reliance on the use of level of performance as a method of inference regarding brain damage is also subject to other frequent misunderstandings. The level of performance on any single measure is not in itself definitive evidence of the presence or absence of a brain lesion. The greater the number of scores and composite indices that are in the range which is characteristic of brain-impaired patients, the more certain one can be that the individual has suffered a brain-impairing event. One should also note that the cut-off scores for the tests of the Halstead-Reitan Battery (Chapter 2) are scores which simply divided groups of patients into those who had demonstrable brain damage and those who did not have such impairments in previous research projects. Russell, Neuringer, and Goldstein (1970), on the other hand, have scaled the scores of the tests in the battery for severity of impairment. Whether one uses the Halstead-Reitan cut-off scores or the Russell et al. (1970) scales, it is important to recognize that the severity of impairment on each score or index should be taken into consideration along with the data showing whether the score is in the "impaired" or "nonimpaired" range.

Two additional factors should be considered in assessing the level of performance on the various test scores and indices of the battery. The first of these is that conditions other than identifiable brain damage can lower scores on many tests of the battery. Assessment of psychiatric patients in particular must be tempered with the fact that conditions which are generally considered functional disorders, such as depression and psychosis, can lower scores. Golden (1977), for example, has shown that the usual cut-off scores for the Halstead-Reitan Battery do not distinguish brain-damaged from intact patients in a psychiatric population as well as they do in a non-psychiatric sample. There is, in fact, growing evidence for a neurochemical and/or metabolic basis for many psychiatric disturbances (e.g., Heaton & Crowley, 1981). The second factor that should be addressed is the fact that some patients with discrete localized brain lesions will perform in the nonimpaired range on many of the tests of the Battery. The implication of this is that the level of performance on tests of the Battery cannot by itself be taken as a definite indication of whether or not a patient has a brain-impairing lesion. In using level of performance as a method of inference the psychologist should consider the scores in relationship to the cut-off scores presented in Chapter 2 and/or the scales shown on the neuropsychological profile form in this chapter.

2) Psychologists have also traditionally used the **pattern of performance** among different test scores as an indication of the presence or absence of brain damage. Matarazzo (1972) for example, reviewed a number of studies in which Verbal IQ-Performance IQ differences were used to infer the presence or absence of brain damage. The Shipley Institute of Living Scale (Shipley, 1940) is one example of a number of other tests that have utilized comparisons of performance on different types of tasks as a means of inferring brain damage. Just as the sole reliance on level of performance as a method of inference will lead to many false conclusions, so will focusing only on interpretation of patterns of test scores.

In the following chapters the reader will find hypotheses regarding the implications of different patterns of test scores. These should be studied in such a way that the most common and most important of them will be obvious on inspection of test data. One of the relationships which illustrates the importance of answering the above questions in a logical sequence relates to the possible effect of lateralized lesions on Verbal – Performance IQ differences. One might mistakenly conclude that a patient has a right cerebral hemisphere lesion because Performance IQ is considerably lower than Verbal IQ, without first addressing the question of whether there is in fact sufficient evidence to conclude that the patient has brain damage.

Some of the other important hypotheses in subsequent chapters relate to interpretation of patterns on test scores such as relationships between the scores on tests such as the Seashore Rhythm Test and Speech-sounds Perception Test. The relationship between the scores on the TPT, for example, and more purely motor tests have implications for anterior or posterior location of lesions. The relationship between the results on the Seashore Rhythm Test and the Speech-sounds Perception Test, on the other hand, may have implications for acuteness and severity of the disorder. It is essential, however, to recognize the strength of the implications of each of these patterns, as well as any other patterns that one may consider.

3) While psychologists have historically tended to rely principally on the above two methods of inference, neurologists have focused more on **differences in the sensory, motor, and reflex functioning of the two sides of the body** to infer the presence and location of brain-impairing lesions. This method of inference results in the strongest implications for lateralization of the lesion. Data on the test battery which lead to this type of inference include the difference in performance of the two hands on the TPT, Finger Oscillation Test, Strength of Grip, and the Sensory Perceptual Examination. Discrepancies between the performance of the two sides of the body which exceed the

normal expectations have very strong implications for lateralization and severity of a lesion.

4) Just as neurologists rely on differences in functioning of the two sides of the body, they also rely on the **presence of pathognomonic signs,** such as the Babinski reflex, in drawing conclusions about neurological disorders. The neuropsychologist also looks for such definitive signs of brain impairment, particularly on the Aphasia Screening Test and on the Sensory Perceptual Examination. The presence of obvious aphasic signs on the Aphasia Screening Test, unilateral suppressions, or visual field defects on the Sensory Perceptual Examination are pathognomonic signs of brain damage, as well as indications of lateralization and sometimes localization.

Answers to the previously discussed critical questions should be attempted by the neuropsychologist using all four methods of inference. Reliance on only one or two of them may result in unfortunate false positive or false negative inferences. Use of level of performance alone, for example, may yield false positive inferences because a number of other factors such as cultural deprivation, educational disadvantage, and various psychiatric conditions, may in turn lead to poor levels of performance on many tests. On the other hand, reliance only on the presence of pathognomonic signs, or differences in functioning of the two sides of the body, may lead to false negative inferences, particularly when there are diffuse, generalized lesions. As Reitan (1967) has suggested, the combination of these four methods of inference is the most powerful way of evaluating neuropsychological test data. When such data are considered from the perspectives of all four methods of inference, one is much less likely to make either false negative or false positive errors.

To summarize, these four methods of inference are complimentary and should be used in combination to interpret neuropsychological test data. In assessing the level of performance, the reader should refer to the section of the Guide on cut-off scores (pg. 19). Patterns of performance on different tests and subtests can be evaluated by referring to the individual test hypotheses. One should look for the presence of pathognomonic signs on the Aphasia Screening Test and the Sensory Perceptual Examination; while differential performance of the two sides of the body can be evaluated by comparing the results of the Sensory Perceptual Examination, Finger Oscillation Test, Strength of Grip, and TPT.

In analyzing neuropsychological test data from the Halstead-Reitan Battery, the use of this Guide should proceed through the following steps and questions as described below.

First, transcribe the neuropsychological test data from the test records themselves or from the data summary sheet such as the one described in Chapter 2 (Figure 3) onto a neuropsychological profile sheet. An example of one useful neuropsychological assessment profile form is shown in Figure 4. This is essentially a hybrid form which utilizes many but not all of the Russell, Neuringer, and Goldstein (1970) scales. It does not, for example, utilize the

FIGURE 4

NEUROPSYCHOLOGICAL ASSESSMENT PROFILE

Patient Name:_____ Age:_____ Sex:_____ Education:_____ Handedness:_____

Rating Equivalents of Raw Scores

Test	0	1	2	3	4	5
Impairment Index	0 ┼ .2 　.3 ┼	.4 　.5 ┼	.6 　.7 ┼	.8 　.9 ┼	1.0	
Category Errors	≤ 25	26-52	53-75	76-105	106-131	132+
(TPT) Time-Dom.	≤ 4.7	4.8-8.2	8.3-10	10 & 9-5 in.	10 & 4-2 in.	10 & 1-0 in.
(TPT) Nondom.	≤ 2.6	2.7-4.5	4.6-6.1	6.2-8.8	8.9-10&10-6 in	10 & 5-0 in.
(TPT) Both	≤ 1.5	1.6-2.7	2.8-3.7	3.8-5.2	5.3-10	10 & 0-9 in.
(TPT) Total	≤ 9.0	9.1-15.6	15.7-21	21.1-29.9	30 & 14-30 in.	30 & 0-13 in
(TPT) Memory	10-9	8-6	5-4	3-2	1	0
(TPT) Localization	10-7	6-5	4-3	2-1	0 & mem > 0	0 & mem = 0
Rhythm Errors	0-2	3-5	6-9	10-13	14-18	19+
Speech Errors	0-3	4-7	8-14	15-25	26-30	31+
Tapping (No.)						
Dom. M	≥ 55	54-50	49-43	42-32	31-20	19-0
F	≥ 51	50-46	45-39	38-28	27-16	15-0
Nondom. M	≥ 49	48-44	43-37	36-26	25-14	13-0
F	≥ 45	44-40	39-33	32-22	21-10	9-0
Trails A (time)	≤ 19	20-33	34-48	49-62	63-86	87+
Trails B (time)	≤ 57	58-87	88-123	124-186	187-275	276+
Memory						
ST	27+	24-26	18-23	14-17	9-13	0-8
(verbal) ½ Hr.	24+	20-23	15-19	9-14	4-8	0-3
% Ret.	99-100	85-98	69-84	51-68	32-50	0-31
ST	12+	10-11	8-9	5-7	2-4	0-1
(figures)½ Hr.	11+	9-11	7-8	4-6	1-3	0
% Ret.	99-100	84-98	66-83	45-65	25-44	0-24

Verbal IQ _____ WMQ_____ Performance IQ _____

From *Assessment of Brain Damage – A Neuropsychological Key Approach* by E. W. Russell, C. Neuringer, and G. Goldstein, New York: Wiley, 1970; and "A multiple scoring method for the assessment of complex motor functions," *Journal of Consulting and Clinical Psychology*, 1975, *43*, 6, 800-809. Copyright 1975 by the American Psychological Association. Reprinted/Adapted by permission of the publishers.

Russell et al. Average Impairment Rating; instead, the Halstead Impairment Index is placed on the top line in the appropriate column. This means that Halstead Impairment Indices .2-.3 are placed under the 1 rating, .4 and .5 are placed under the 2 rating, .6 and .7 under the 3 rating, .8 and .9 under the 4 rating, and 1.0 under the 5 rating. Scores from other tests in the battery are placed in the appropriate box on each line. It will quickly be seen in using this form that a "profile" is readily obtained which offers a general indication of **degree of impairment** in various functional areas as well as facilitating comparison of scores on different tests in order to make possible inferences regarding patterns of test scores. As indicated earlier, it is more difficult to make such inferences if one only uses Reitan's cut-off scores to divide patients into two groups – brain-damaged and intact.

The next step is to address each of the critical questions using the four methods of inference. The hypotheses used in this process are presented in Chapters 4-7, and illustrations of the process are provided in Chapter 11.

QUESTIONS TO BE ANSWERED

1) Is there cerebral impairment?
Level of Performance – The scores on all tests should be compared with the cut-off scores (pg. 22) for brain damage, with special attention paid to those tests most sensitive to cerebral impairment. The hypotheses in Chapter 4 are most important here.

Pattern of Performance – The relevant hypotheses in Chapter 4 should be checked for relationships shown on the profile which are deviant from normal expectations. The hypotheses regarding the WAIS scores are particularly important here.

Right-Left Differences – The performance on the TPT, Finger Oscillation, and Strength of Grip Tests, and the difference in performance of the two sides of the body on the Sensory Perceptual Examination should all be checked for deviations from the expected performance. Such deviations have relevance for this question as well as the later one regarding lateralization.

Pathognomonic Signs – Hypotheses regarding these signs will be found among those related to the Aphasia Screening Test and the Sensory Perceptual Examination. The presence of any such signs in the data is a strong argument for an affirmative answer to this question in regard to the presence or absence of brain damage.

2) What is the severity of the damage?
Level of Performance – The pattern of the scores on the profile sheet should be examined in terms of the degree of impairment on each of the tests. Particular attention should be paid to those tests which are most sensitive to impairment and to those which represent functions most important to the patient being examined.

Pattern of Performance – Here it is the magnitude of the deviation from expected patterns of performance that is most relevant regarding the question of severity. A particular relationship must be considered in the context of each individual patient. For example, a Verbal IQ 15 points below a Performance IQ has different implications for an attorney than for a mechanic.

Right-Left Differences – Once again the magnitude of the difference from expected performance is the key factor in assessing severity.

Pathognomonic Signs – Generally, the presence of any pathognomonic sign indicates definite impairment and, of course, a greater number of such signs suggests greater severity.

3) Is the lesion progressive or static?

Level of Performance – The hypotheses regarding specific tests in Chapter 4 should be checked for indications regarding velocity. One should note that it is often possible to state with more confidence that a lesion is relatively static than that it is progressive. For example, adequate performance on the Seashore Rhythm and Speech-sounds Perception Tests makes a progressive lesion less likely, but poor performance on these tests can result from factors other than a progressive lesion.

Pattern of Performance – The hypotheses related to WAIS performance in Chapter 4 are the most relevant ones regarding this question.

Right-Left Differences – This method of inference does not usually yield useful information regarding this question.

Pathognomonic Signs – Certain pathognomonic signs are frequently seen in cases with rapidly progressive lesions, but one should note that they may still be present, if there has been actual tissue destruction, even after a lesion has become static and chronic.

4) Is the lesion diffuse or lateralized?

Level of Performance – This method of inference does not yield information relevant to this question.

Pattern of Performance – The hypotheses in Chapter 4 should be checked against the data for lateralizing signs. One should note, however, that the lateralizing signs seen in patterns of performance are all relatively weak ones.

Right-Left Differences – This is the method of inference that is most useful in answering the question of diffuse vs. lateralized lesions. Differences in the performance on the two sides of the body should be checked carefully on the TPT, Finger Oscillation Test, Strength of Grip, and Sensory Perceptual Examination.

Pathognomonic Signs – Pathognomonic signs, which may be found on the Aphasia Screening Test and Sensory Perceptual Examination, are also among the most powerful indicators of lateralization.

5) Is the impairment in the anterior or posterior portion of the cerebral hemisphere?

Level of Performance – This method of inference does not yield information relevant to this question.

Pattern of Performance – The most useful patterns of performance to be considered are those described in the hypotheses relating performance on motor tasks to performance on sensory tasks. Other hypotheses regarding patterns of WAIS subtest scores (e.g., BD-PA) and constructional dyspraxia should also be considered.

Right-Left Differences – This method of inference does not yield information relevant to this question.

Pathognomonic Signs – Some pathognomonic signs may have very specific implications for localization, and the hypotheses related to any such signs should be checked carefully. Visual field defects are a prime example.

6) What is the most likely neuropathological process?

The answer to this question is based first on a review of the answers to the preceding five questions. On this basis one can first determine which broad neuropathological category must be considered. For example, if a diffuse, slowly progressive lesion is involved, the focus must be on the degenerative or infectious processes. On the other hand, if a highly lateralized, acute, or progressive picture is presented, the destructive neoplastic and vascular conditions should be considered. Once such a general process category has been identified, it is necessary to review the specific hypotheses related to all of the individual possibilities within that category as described in Chapter 7. In this way, fairly accurate answers can frequently be formulated for this question. This can be a very intriguing result. It is important to remember, however, that this is not the most important function of the neuropsychologist.

7) What are the implications for daily functioning and treatment?

Although the bulk of this Guide has been aimed at teaching a method for answering the preceding six questions, it is in answering this seventh question that the neuropsychologist makes a unique and most important contribution.

The patient's performance on the tests in the battery provides the neuropsychologist with a sample of the abilities required for everyday activities. In order to generalize from this sample or to predict functioning in other activities, the requirements for performance of the tests described in Chapter 2 must be considered. It is also important to evaluate both the strengths and weaknesses shown by the patient.

Of particular concern to the neuropsychologist is prediction of functioning in three general areas: self-care, management of one's personal affairs, and school or work activities. The ability to care for one's self and live relatively independently requires at the very minimum adequate motor abilities and sensory functioning. The more independently one lives, the greater the need for additional abilities. These include attention, concentration, memory, the ability to follow directions, and communication and problem solving skills. The potential living arrangements for each patient must be analyzed in terms of their requirements for these skills, and the patient's strengths and weaknesses compared to these requirements.

Assessment of ability to manage one's own affairs depends on the complexity of the patient's personal situation. In addition to adequate abilities in all of the areas required for self-care, higher levels of functioning are usually required in communication, memory, and problem solving (as well as adequate skills in reading, arithmetic, awareness of current events, and general information).

The ability to function at work or in school will have requirements that vary tremendously with the nature of the job or studies, and these requirements must be considered in relationship to the patient's cognitive and behavioral strengths and weaknesses. Occasionally, changes in vocation or course of study will be indicated in order to maximize the possibility of success.

Heaton and Pendleton (1981) have provided a number of additional suggestions regarding possible implications of performance on specific tests for everyday functioning. It is also important to keep in mind three general principles in planning treatment: 1) build on the patient's demonstrated strengths, 2) compensate for weaknesses by teaching alternative methods of accomplishing tasks, and 3) provide retraining for impaired skills. Factors such as the patient's awareness of deficits and his or her reaction to them as well as the reactions and expectations of other people (discussed in Chapter 8), must also be considered in treatment planning.

CAVEAT

While it is hoped that this Guide will be an aid, particularly for psychologists in mental health settings, to the better understanding of and cautious interpretation of neuropsychological test data on adult patients, it must be emphasized that users not overextend the limits of this Guide and their formal training. Some of the developments in the field of clinical neuropsychology have been dramatic and one may be tempted to make highly specific diagnoses or predictions about the location and nature of brain lesions. To do so, however, without a high level of accuracy, will not only decrease the credibility of the individual practitioner and the entire profession, but more importantly, will do grave disservice to many patients. It is to these concerns that this CAVEAT is addressed.

By now many psychologists have been exposed to the extremely detailed and usually accurate interpretation that experts such as Reitan can make from standardized test battery data. Furthermore, Goldstein, Daysack, and Kleinknecht (1973) have demonstrated that psychology interns can be trained in a relatively short period of time to make valid identifications of the presence of brain damage using the Halstead-Reitan Battery. One must remember, however, that the predictions made by the subjects in the Goldstein et al. study were not as detailed as the predictions made by many of the experts in the field. It is also important for the clinical psychologist working in the typical mental health setting to remember that Reitan and his associates have worked primarily in neurosurgical departments of medical schools. In these settings they were dealing with very different populations than those with which most psychologists in the typical clinical settings are faced. Also, it is important to remember that they had exposure to thousands of cases of demonstrated brain damage. This Guide is in no way intended to substitute for this type of vast experience.

There are other problems in making highly refined diagnoses and specific statements regarding localization of lesions that some psychologists may have overlooked. The first of these is that many of our anatomical descriptions are quite general. Meyer, quoting Bailey (1955), states, "It must be realized that the various regions of the brain do not constitute functional subdivisions in any sense. The lobes were originally named after the cranial bones under which they lie and as such represent a crude anatomical classification" (1961, p. 555).

A further complication of this general "map" of the cortex stems from the nature and effect of the pathological lesions with which we are dealing. Any lesion, whether due to atrophy, tumor, or trauma, does not affect a clearly limited area of the brain and the functions mediated by that area. Instead, it exerts effects through disruption of blood supply, pressure effects on other parts of the brain, and disruptions of connections between various areas of the cerebral hemispheres. Surgical intervention can have similar effects, although in many of these cases there remains considerable uncertainty as to the extent of pathology in portions of the brain which were not directly exposed during surgery. Another factor limiting even the work of Reitan and others who have been involved in his tradition with neurosurgical patients is that it is frequently not possible to obtain definite information about either the premorbid condition of the brain or the premorbid functioning of the patient. This factor is certainly more significant to psychologists working in a mental health setting where this evidence is even more difficult to obtain in a way that would permit detailed comparison with current performance on a complex neuropsychological test battery.

As a final word in this admonitory section, it must be stressed again that the psychologist in most mental health settings seldom sees the "clean" cases on which the Halstead-Reitan Battery research was developed. Instead, one is more likely to see a 60-year-old chronic alcoholic patient who has incurred multiple head injuries while intoxicated, suffers from malnutrition and has been institutionalized for a long period of time either in a "traditional institution" or in one of the newer community settings. There is frequently little reliable medical or social history available and there are few cues from the fragmentary vocational background as to the patient's premorbid or optimal level of functioning in almost any area. If this is not complicated enough, the patient may be psychotic at times and the referral question may be "Please differentiate organicity from schizophrenia or other psychosis." While this case is extreme, it is not uncommon, and many such referrals present several if not all of the above complications. This illustrates the difficulties and dangers of extrapolating from clean neurosurgical cases to the complex realities of life of many practicing clinical psychologists.

The reader should also note that this Guide addresses only the neuropsychological evaluation of adult patients. While there is a growing body of literature in the field of clinical neuropsychology of children, results are generally not as clear cut and one should not attempt to extrapolate totally from the hypotheses or inferences included here to the assessment of children.

It is hoped that these cautionary statements will prompt the reader not to overdiagnose or make unequivocal statements about the presence or absence of brain damage, and not to formulate rash predictions concerning the location and nature of brain pathology. It is instead hoped that this Guide will be a useful tool in understanding and interpreting neuropsychological test data and that it will aid in formulating more useful treatment plans for patients.

Chapter 4

TEST HYPOTHESES

IMPAIRMENT INDEX

As indicated earlier, the Halstead Impairment Index is a composite measure of the level of performance on the tests of the Halstead-Reitan Battery. It simply indicates the proportion of those test scores which are in the range characteristic of brain-impaired patients; therefore, all of the considerations regarding interpretation of level of performance indicators identified in Chapter 2 should be observed in evaluating the Impairment Index. One should also note that this Index tends to be correlated to some extent with intelligence and that the significance of an elevated Impairment Index decreases with age, as indicated below. Taking these factors into consideration, however, the Impairment Index is still the most sensitive indicator of brain impairment.

While the level of the Impairment Index is often interpreted as an indicator of the severity of brain damage, one needs to recognize that it is possible to have an Impairment Index of 1.0 (all of the tests in the battery in the impaired range) with only a mild degree of impairment. For example, if a patient has 52 errors on the Category Test; scores on the TPT of 16 minutes total time, memory-5 and localization-4; 24 items correct on the Seashore Rhythm Test; 14 errors on the Speech-sounds Perception Test; and a Finger Tapping score of 50 with the dominant hand, he or she would have an Impairment Index of 1.0. Since each of these scores is just barely in the impaired range, however, it should be clear that the overall impairment is mild even though all of the scores fall above the cut-off points. The Average Impairment Rating of Russell, Neuringer, and Goldstein (1970) takes this factor into consideration, and one may either use the Average Impairment Rating or examine each of the individual scores, as well as the overall Impairment Index, in making a judgment about the degree of severity of impairment.

(4-1) The most sensitive general indicators of brain impairment (level of performance scores) are: 1) Impairment Index, 2) Category, 3) TPT Localization, and 4) Trails B, in that order of sensitivity (Reitan, 1959).

(4-2) The significance of an elevated Impairment Index decreases with age after age 45-50.

(4-3) Prognosis for recovery of language functions is relatively good even with clear-cut indications of left cerebral hemisphere damage if the Impairment Index is relatively low and certain other scores such as Category, Speech-sounds Perception, and Seashore Rhythm are adequate.

(4-4) The validity of the Impairment Index as an indicator of brain damage appears to be greater when the IQ falls within the normal range or above.

(4-5) Patients with Parkinson's disease often perform poorly on the Category Test, tend to have relatively high impairment indices, and perform poorly on Trail Making; their IQs may be in the average range (Reitan & Boll, 1971).

(4-6) An intact IQ and an Impairment Index above .5 suggest significant brain damage.

(4-7) The Impairment Index tends to be higher in cases with tissue destruction such as intracerebral neoplasms, CVAs, and penetrating head injuries, and may be lower in cases of extracerebral neoplasms and mild to moderate closed head injuries (Golden, 1978).

WAIS

The Full Scale IQ on the Wechsler Adult Intelligence Scale, when viewed from the perspective of level of performance, is primarily useful when it is compared to other data. Previous performance on this same test is the best comparative data to determine whether there is an overall deterioration in intellectual functioning. Many times previous testing is not available, however, and one must use estimates of previous level of intellectual functioning such as educational and vocational background. A person with a college degree and a vocational history consistent with his or her education, for example, who achieves a Full Scale IQ of 80 is demonstrating a significant level of impairment whether this is due to identifiable brain damage or a psychiatric condition.

The data from the WAIS, however, should also be considered in terms of the pattern of scores on the Verbal IQ, Performance IQ, and the individual subtests. The hypotheses in this section indicate a number of important relationships among scores. The pattern of subtest scores often yields valuable information about strengths and weaknesses that may be useful in planning rehabilitation programs.

(4-8) An intact IQ and an Impairment Index above .5 suggest significant brain damage.

(4-9) In a brain-damaged person with a high level of education, a low IQ score suggests that the impairment is severe.

(4-10) IQ tends to be negatively correlated with Category scores (Cullum, Steinman, & Bigler, 1984).

(4-11) If there is a good indication of brain damage, yet IQ scores are relatively unimpaired, a static lesion is suggested.

(4-12) Patients with Parkinson's disease often perform poorly on the Category Test, tend to have relatively high impairment indices, and perform poorly on Trail Making; their IQs may be in the average range (Reitan & Boll, 1971).

(4-13) Closed head injuries can produce mild and often diffuse damage which may not significantly affect Full Scale IQ or create a difference between VIQ and PIQ. With this type of pathology one may see mixed signs or different levels of impairment because of the contrecoup and shear/strain effects.

VIQ – PIQ DIFFERENCES

(4-14) When Performance IQ is 20 or more points lower than Verbal IQ on the WAIS, this suggests the possibility of right cerebral hemisphere damage. When the reverse is true, left cerebral hemisphere damage is suspected. One must temper this finding with the fact that the Performance IQ is more likely to be affected by a cerebral lesion than is Verbal IQ due to the fact that the Performance subtests involve new and unique learning; Verbal subtests measure accumulated knowledge which is the least affected by brain damage.

(4-15) Extracerebral tumors rarely result in signficant VIQ-PIQ differences.

(4-16) Localizing or lateralizing signs in the *absence* of depressed FSIQ and with little PIQ – VIQ difference suggest the *absence* of intracerebral tumor or vascular disorder.

(4-17) No significant difference between Verbal and Performance IQ suggests either diffuse damage or a static (or slowly progressive) lesion (Reitan, 1959).

(4-18) When there are definite indications of left cerebral hemisphere damage such as dysphasia and lower Verbal IQ, but no indication of left cerebral hemisphere signs on TPT and Tapping, a focal lesion located at some distance from the motor strip is suggested (Reitan, 1959).

WAIS SUBTESTS

Similarities

(4-19) A very low score on Similarities suggests left temporal lobe damage. A normal Similiarities score, however, does not suggest the absence of left temporal lobe damage (Reitan, 1959).

Block Design – Picture Arrangement

(4-20) A Block Design score significantly lower than the Picture Arrangement score suggests a (right) parietal-occipital lesion; a Picture Arrangement score lower than the Block Design score suggests a (right) anterior temporal lobe lesion (Reitan, 1959).

(4-21) If Picture Arrangement and Block Design scores are both depressed, a right temporal-parietal lesion is suggested (Reitan, 1959).

Digit Symbol

(4-22) One of the most sensitive general indicators of brain damage is Digit Symbol, provided there are other signs of impairment on the Halstead-Reitan Battery (Golden, 1978).

Digit Span

(4-23) Many hospitalized patients show a low score on Digit Span; therefore, this is one of the poorest predictors of identifiable brain damage.

Information – Vocabulary

(4-24) The Information and Vocabulary subtests from the WAIS are less susceptible to brain damage than other subtest scores; therefore, they may offer an indication of premorbid functioning (Golden, 1978).

CATEGORY TEST

As indicated, the Category Test is the single test most sensitive to damage to any area of the brain. Occasionally, however, one will see a patient with demonstrable brain damage who performs quite well on this test. One young man, for example, who had suffered a severe closed head injury, performed very well on the Category Test, making only 14 errors. This is an exceptionally good score on this test for a person with his education (12 years) and IQ (Full Scale IQ-114). This level of performance obviously has major implications for the rehabilitation of this man who has severe motor and sensory impairments due to his injury.

(4-25) The most sensitive general indicators of brain damage (level of performance scores) are: 1) Impairment Index, 2) Category, 3) TPT Localization, and 4) Trails B (Reitan, 1959).

(4-26) IQ tends to be negatively correlated with Category scores (Cullum, Steinman, & Bigler, 1984).

(4-27) If scores on both Category and Part B of Trail Making are poor, while other tests are near normal, a focal and static lesion of one or both anterior frontal lobes may be suggested (Reitan, 1959).

(4-28) Adequate performance on the Category Test even in the presence of a high Impairment Index and poor performance on other tests does not appear consistent with either intracerebral tumors or massive CVAs, since damage of this type usually impairs abstraction ability regardless of the location of the lesion.

(4-29) Prognosis for recovery of language functions is relatively good even with clear-cut indications of left cerebral hemisphere damage if the Impairment Index is relatively low and certain other scores such as Category, Speech-sounds Perception, and Seashore Rhythm are in the normal range.

(4-30) Patients with Parkinson's disease often perform poorly on the Category Test and Trail Making and tend to have relatively high impairment indices; their IQs may be in the average range (Reitan & Boll, 1971).

(4-31) Alcoholics do most poorly on the Category Test and show overall low scores across the entire battery.

TRAIL MAKING TEST

The Trail Making Test, particularly Part B, is one of the more sensitive general indicators of brain damage. The score on Part B may also have implications for certain aspects of the patient's daily functioning. For example, a particularly poor score on Part B indicates that the patient has difficulty in following complex patterns of visual stimuli involving alternation between two sets of symbols. This may suggest (particularly if scores on other tests which have similar requirements are low) that the patient will have difficulty in driving an automobile in strange territory and heavy traffic.

One of the hypotheses in this section indicates that the difference between the scores on Part A and Part B on the Trail Making Test may have some implications for lateralization to one cerebral hemisphere or the other. It should be noted, however, that the implication of this difference for lateralization is not a strong one, and inferences about lateralization of a lesion should never be based on this relationship alone.

(4-32) The most sensitive general indicators of level of brain damage (performance scores) are: 1) Impairment Index, 2) Category, 3) TPT Localization, and 4) Trails B, in that order of significance (Reitan, 1959).

(4-33) A score on Trails B which is substantially poorer than the score on Trails A suggests left hemisphere damage, while a lower score on Part A suggests right cerebral hemisphere damage. This is a weak hypothesis unless substantiated by other data (Reitan & Tarshes, 1959).

(4-34) If scores on both Category and Part B of Trail Making are poor while other tests are near normal, a focal and static lesion of one or both anterior frontal lobes may be suggested (Reitan, 1959).

(4-35) Patients with Parkinson's disease often perform poorly on the Category Test, tend to have relatively high impairment indices, and perform poorly on Trail Making; their IQs may be in the average range (Reitan & Boll, 1971).

TACTUAL PERFORMANCE TEST

While the localization score on the TPT is one of the more sensitive general indicators of brain damage, the most valuable information derived from the scores on this test is the difference in performance between the dominant and nondominant hands. As indicated in the following hypotheses, this has strong implications for lateralization of lesions.

Since the TPT is a test with very complex requirements for satisfactory performance, having both motor and sensory components, it is important to compare the scores on this test with those on other tests which have some (but not all) of the same requirements that the TPT does. For example, it is often useful to compare performance on the TPT with test results from Finger Oscillation, which has only simple motor speed requirements. This, of course, has implications for location of the lesion more anteriorly or posteriorly, depending on which test score is more impaired. If one were to use only the Halstead-Reitan cut-off scores, such a comparison would be difficult. It is more useful to use the scales developed by Russell et al. (1970) or a profile sheet in making such comparisons.

There is an expected relationship between the performance of the two hands on the TPT due to intracerebral transfer of information and learning effects. The time with the dominant hand (which is always tested first) should be greatest (e.g., 3-5 minutes), while the time with the nondominant hand should be less (e.g., 2-3 minutes) and the time with both hands should be lowest (e.g., 1-3 minutes). Any deviation from these expectations strongly suggests lateralization of a lesion. For example, in a right-handed patient, if the time with the left hand (second trial) is greater than the time with the right hand, this has strong implications for lateralization of a lesion to the contra-lateral (right) hemisphere. Lateralization in this direction is most obvious when the nondominant hand is actually slower.

Somewhat more subtle, however, are those cases in which the nondom-inant hand is faster than the dominant hand, but where the difference is not as great as one would expect. The expectation is that there should be about a 30% improvement from one trial to the next. Consider, for example, a patient whose time with the dominant hand is 8.0 minutes and whose time with the nondominant hand is 6.5 minutes. This represents an improvement of less than 20% and suggests lateralization to the cerebral hemisphere contralateral to the nondominant hand. This can be seen very readily without calculating the percentage of improvement by locating those times on the same profile sheet in Chapter 3. When one does this, it is readily apparent that the non-dominant hand is more impaired. (The time for the dominant hand gets a score of 1 and the time for the nondominant hand gets a score of 3.)

Another subtle case is the one in which there is "too much" improvement between the first and second trials. Consider the example of the patient who places nine blocks correctly in ten minutes with the dominant hand, but is able to place all ten blocks correctly in four minutes with the nondominant hand. This is an improvement of more than 60%. Once again, the lateralization effect is immediately obvious if one locates these scores on the profile sheet which shows a score of 3 for the dominant hand and a score of 1 for the nondominant hand.

Regardless of which of the first two trials was better, one should consider the time on the third trial (with both hands). The time on this trial should be less than the time on the faster of the first two trials. When it is not, or when the difference does not reach the expected degree of improvement, this sug-gests that the more impaired hand is actually interfering with the performance of the other hand when both are used. This is an indication of severe impair-ment which is often seen in patients with significant tissue-destroying lesions such as intracerebral neoplasms. An example of this would be a patient who only placed 7 blocks correctly in ten minutes with the dominant hand, placed all 10 blocks correctly with the nondominant hand in 5 minutes and placed all ten blocks correctly with both hands in 4.5 minutes. Locating these times on the profile sheet shows scores of 3 for the dominant hand, 2 for the nondom-inant hand, and 3 for both hands; thus the dominant right hand (left cerebral hemisphere) interference effect is obvious.

Finally, one may sometimes encounter cases in which the performance gets steadily slower as the trials progress. In such cases, particularly if the number of blocks placed correctly also decreases with each succeeding trial, fatigue may be a factor. If this is the case, there should be supporting data seen on other motor tests and in general observations of the patient's performance.

Another hypothesis which may need to be considered, particularly in psychiatric populations, is that the patient is becoming more resistant, less motivated, or depressed over perceived failures as testing progresses. Evaluation of these hypotheses is aided by careful observation and recording of the patient's cooperation, effort, and general approach to the testing situation.

> **(4-36)** The most sensitive general indicators of brain damage (performance scores) are: 1) Impairment Index, 2) Category, 3) TPT Localization, and 4) Trails B, in that order of significance (Reitan, 1959).

> **(4-37)** Reversal of TPT relationships becomes more common and less significant with increasing age, because fatigue becomes a more important factor.

> **(4-38)** If TPT performance is more impaired than Finger Oscillation performance with the same hand, a posterior lesion is suggested, i.e., at some distance from the motor strip. If Finger Oscillation is more impaired than TPT with the same hand, a lesion in the anterior part of the contralateral hemisphere is suggested (Reitan, 1959).

> **(4-39)** When there are definite indications of left cerebral hemisphere damage such as dysphasia and lowered Verbal IQ, but no indication of left cerebral hemisphere signs on TPT and Finger Oscillation, this suggests a focal lesion located at some distance from the motor strip (Reitan, 1959).

SEASHORE RHYTHM TEST

As indicated in Chapter 2. the Seashore Rhythm Test is not simply a test of auditory discrimination of different patterns of rhythms; instead, it has complex attention and concentration requirements for satisfactory performance. It is important to determine just which of these requirements the patient was not able to meet satisfactorily in order to interpret the score most accurately on the Seashore Rhythm Test. Precise information about how the patient performed or failed to perform adequately on this test is important, and a second trial on the test with modified requirements for performance may supply additional information. (See Chapter 1 for further suggestions about modifications that may be useful.)

One should note that the indication of possible lateralization of a lesion derived from the relationship between the score on this test and the score on the Speech-sounds Perception Test is a weak one and should not by itself be taken as a true indication of lateralization of a lesion.

(4-40) Adequate scores on the Speech-sounds Perception Test and the Seashore Rhythm Test indicate that there probably is *not* a rapidly progressive lesion. These scores are also good measures of recovery following a CVA or trauma.

(4-41) Very poor Seashore Rhythm and Speech-sounds Perception scores may suggest general destruction of brain tissue (Golden, 1978).

(4-42) If aphasic signs are present and Speech-sounds Perception and Seashore Rhythm scores are depressed, a left temporal lesion may be suspected.

(4-43) A very low score on the Speech-sounds Perception Test in relation to the score on the Seashore Rhythm Test may suggest left hemisphere damage; the reverse suggests right hemisphere damage, although these are weak signs by themselves.

SPEECH-SOUNDS PERCEPTION TEST

The comments in the preceding section on the Seashore Rhythm Test generally apply to interpretations of the Speech-sounds Perception Test and will not be repeated here.

FINGER OSCILLATION TEST

The level of performance on this test is a relatively weak indicator of brain damage since there is a wide range of scores achieved by both brain-damaged and intact patients. On the other hand, a difference in the performances of the dominant and nondominant hands is a strong indicator of lateralization of lesion. As indicated above, it is often useful to compare performance on this test with performance on other tests, such as the TPT, in drawing inferences about anterior versus posterior location of a lesion.

Just as performance on the TPT must be interpreted in the light of the expected relationship between the performances of the two hands, so must performance on Finger Oscillation. In this case, however, there is no learning effect to consider and the expectation is simply that the dominant hand will be able to tap about 10% faster than the nondominant hand.

If the dominant hand is not approximately 10% faster than the nondominant hand, a lesion in the hemisphere contralateral to the dominant hand should be suspected. Similarly, if the nondominant hand is considerably more than 10% slower than the dominant hand, a lesion in the hemisphere contralateral to the nondominant hand should be suspected.

(4-44) Retention of simple motor function (tapping speed) in the presence of other severe deficits is sometimes seen in cases of extracerebral neoplasms.

(4-45) If TPT performance is more impaired than Finger Oscillation with the same hand, a posterior lesion in the contralateral hemisphere is suggested, specifically at some distance from the motor strip. If Finger Oscillation is more impaired than TPT with the same hand, a lesion in the anterior part of the contralateral hemisphere is suspected (Reitan, 1959).

(4-46) When there are definite indications of left cerebral hemisphere damage such as dysphasia and lowered Verbal IQ, but no indication of left cerebral hemisphere signs on TPT and Finger Oscillation, a focal lesion located at some distance from the motor strip is suggested (Reitan, 1959).

(4-47) Definite sex differences are apparent on both Finger Oscillation and Strength of Grip. (A score of 15-20 kilograms is generally expected for most females on the Hand Dynamometer, whereas 40-50 kilograms is expected for most males). Finger Oscillation scores for females should be slightly slower (10%) than for males. Other subtests of the Halstead-Reitan Neuropsychological Test Battery should not be affected by sex differences.

(4-48) If motor functions such as tapping and strength of grip are depressed, one would expect a lesion in the anterior part of the brain near the motor strip.

(4-49) If Finger Oscillation scores are vastly different (e.g., dominant-3, nondominant-49), a cardiovascular accident is suspected. A head injury or tumor can probably be ruled out due to the fact that it would have done more damage to the other cerebral hemisphere.

(4-50) If TPT scores are depressed and Finger Oscillation is within normal limits, this suggests sensory strip involvement (Reitan, 1959).

STRENGTH OF GRIP (HAND DYNAMOMETER)

Scores on the Strength of Grip may have definite implications for lateralization of cerebral lesions. In interpreting Hand Dynamometer scores, one needs to take into consideration not only sex differences, but also age, physical activity, and occupation. A low score, for example, would be more significant in a young male patient who had previously engaged in heavy manual labor than it would be in an older patient who had engaged only in relatively sedentary occupations and little other physical activity requiring the use of his hands. In general, the hypotheses regarding Finger Oscillation speed also apply to Strength of Grip since both are basically simple motor tests designed to measure right-left differences (10% difference expected between dominant and nondominant upper extremities).

APHASIA SCREENING TEST

The Reitan Indiana Aphasia Screening Test, which is part of the Halstead-Reitan Battery, does not contribute to the Halstead Impairment Index, and is a general screening examination rather than a thorough assessment of all possible aphasic disorders. Nevertheless, pathognomonic signs elicited by this examination are quite significant.

It is important in administering the Aphasia Screening Test to make a verbatim recording of everything that the patient says in response to the questions and instructions. This may help later in distinguishing between true aphasic signs and signs of thought disorder. A verbatim recording will also often assist in detecting mild dysphasic signs that would otherwise go unnoticed if the examiner simply recorded the correct response which was given following several false starts. A common example of this is the patient who responds to the stimulus picture of a fork in a halting manner with "*sp sp sp fork,*" or the patient who responds to the stimulus picture of a Greek cross by saying, "*ah ah ah red cross ahhh cross.*" Such false starts in identifying the stimulus may represent mild dysphasic signs resulting from certain left cerebral hemisphere lesions.

It is important to distinguish between educational deficits and dysphasic signs. The use of the Aphasia Screening Test assumes at least a fourth grade reading level with the significance of dysphasic signs increasing as educational level increases. For example, if a patient spells SQUARE as "SQUAR," (particularly if he/she has a limited education), this may reflect an educational deficit, while spelling it "SQU" may be a dysphasic error. Similarly, the spelling of CROSS as "CROSSSS" is a dysphasic error, especially if it is done by a patient with a twelfth grade education. When one can assume an adequate education, the presence of two or more definite dysphasic errors strongly suggests brain damage.

(**4-51**) Aphasic signs are among the strongest indicators of left cerebral hemisphere damage (Reitan, 1959).

(**4-52**) Dysnomia, dyslexia, dysgraphia, spelling dyspraxia, and dyscalculia, in order of significance, suggest left hemisphere damage. Constructional dyspraxia usually suggests right hemisphere damage. It is important to recognize, however, that 15-20% of subjects who show constructional dyspraxia have left cerebral hemisphere damage only. This is, therefore, a relatively weak lateralizing sign (Reitan, 1959).

(**4-53**) When there are definite indications of left cerebral hemisphere damage such as dysphasia and lowered Verbal IQ but normal scores on TPT and Finger Oscillation, a focal lesion located at some distance from the motor strip is suggested.

(4-54) Expressive aphasic signs, dysnomia, spelling dyspraxia, and dysgraphia suggest left anterior impairment (Reitan, 1959).

(4-55) Receptive aphasic signs, visual form agnosia, visual letter agnosia, dyslexia, auditory verbal agnosia, and auditory number agnosia suggest left posterior impairment. It should be noted that determination of whether certain dysphasic problems are expressive or receptive in nature may require a more thorough aphasia examination than the brief one which is typically part of the battery (Reitan, 1959).

(4-56) If constructional dyspraxia is evident and Block Design is much lower than Picture Arrangement, a right parietal lesion is suggested.

There are certain other relatively infrequent deviant responses on this test which should be noted. These include the following:

(4-57) An attempt to draw the clock instead of writing the word for it as instructed may be a sign of left hemisphere damage.

(4-58) Central dysarthria suggests left hemisphere damage, while slurring may reflect a peripheral problem.

(4-59) If a patient with an adequate education *adds* 85 and 27 instead of subtracting, this may indicate damage to the left cerebral hemisphere and is considered a dyscalculia.

(4-60) Some patients may be unable to demonstrate the use of the key without actually having a key in their hand. This is called ideokinetic dyspraxia and suggests the presence of brain damage.

(4-61) Most patients read the stimulus 7 SIX 2 as "7-6-2." When a patient reads it as "7-S-I-X-2," left hemisphere damage may be suggested.

(4-62) Ignoring the left side of a stimulus, as in responding "6-2" to the stimulus 7 SIX 2, suggests a right parietal lesion. This appears to occur most frequently with patients having destructive lesions such as CVAs or intracerebral neoplasms.

(4-63) Rotation of the key drawing has no significance for brain damage since controls rotate as often as brain-damaged patients.

(4-64) In relatively young adult patients with otherwise healthy brains, impaired language functions appear to improve rapidly; therefore, absence of aphasic symptoms in a young patient with a closed head injury does not rule out trauma to the left side of the brain.

SENSORY PERCEPTUAL EXAMINATION

The most useful data from the Sensory Perceptual Examination are those which show the differential functioning of the right and left sides of the body. Major differences in performance of the two sides of the body are among the stronger indicators of lateralized lesions.

Special note should be made of the performance of some severely impaired patients on the fingertip number writing task. Some people, whether their impairment in functioning is due to a brain lesion or to a psychiatric disturbance, may show many errors on both hands. These multiple errors on both hands are often due to confusion or difficulty in understanding the instructions, particularly when the patient reports numbers which were not included in the instructions. Such errors may have little to do with impaired tactile sensation, particularly when there are no similar errors on other related tasks such as finger agnosia, tactile coin recognition, and tactile form recognition. Readministration of this part of the examination using "X"s and "O"s is often indicated.

(4-65) Visual suppressions suggest damage in the contralateral hemisphere.

(4-66) Visual field defects suggest parietal or temporal lobe damage, often from an intracerebral neoplasm.

(4-67) Loss of sight in one eye suggests damage anterior to the optic chiasm, often from an extracerebral neoplasm or from a peripheral lesion affecting the eye itself.

(4-68) A lesion near the optic chiasm may result in one blind eye and one eye with half field loss. This is sometimes seen in cases with pituitary tumors.

(4-69) Suppressions seldom occur in nonimpaired populations.

(4-70) The absence of any suppression suggests the absence of an acutely destructive space occupying lesion in the posterior part of the cerebral hemisphere (Reitan, 1959).

(4-71) Auditory suppressions suggest damage in the contralateral temporal lobe (Reitan, 1959).

(4-72) Tactile perception is related primarily to parietal lobe functioning; poor scores on fingertip writing, finger agnosia, tactile coin recognition, and tactual form recognition suggest parietal lesions.

(4-73) Misidentification of the circle on the tactile form recognition test is the most serious error on that test.

(4-74) Patients with multiple sclerosis will often show both weakness and transient or spotty sensory perceptual deficits.

(4-75) Severe motor and sensory perceptual loss on one side may be associated with either a rapidly progressive intracerebral neoplasm or more likely an acute cerebral vascular disorder.

(4-76) Sensory suppressions are often associated with cerebrovascular disorders.

Chapter 5

LATERALIZATION AND LOCALIZATION HYPOTHESES

DIFFUSE IMPAIRMENT

Diffuse impairment most often results from degenerative processes such as cortical atrophy, cerebral arterial sclerosis, or infectious diseases such as meningitis. Closed head injuries will often show diffuse impairment but may also exhibit focal signs in the area of greatest trauma. Cases with diffuse impairment must be distinguished from those with multiple localizing signs. With diffuse impairment, if there are motor or sensory deficits on one side of the body, there will usually be similar deficits shown on the other side of the body. In cases of diffuse impairment there will usually be deficits in many functional areas with relatively few areas of cognitive/behavioral functioning remaining intact. In cases with multiple localizing signs, on the other hand, the test battery profile is more varied. If there are motor or sensory deficits on one side of the body, for example, functioning on the other side may be relatively well preserved. Similarly, while many functions may be impaired, others may remain relatively intact. Implications for the most likely pathological process are quite different for these two profiles.

(5-1) The absence of lateralizing signs suggests diffuse impairment (Golden, 1978).

(5-2) No significant difference between Verbal and Performance IQ suggests either diffuse damage or a very old static lesion (Reitan, 1959).

(5-3) Clear, sharp focal deficits and mild to severe generalized damage are sometimes seen with penetrating head injuries (Golden, 1978).

53

(5-4) Very poor Seashore Rhythm and Speech-sounds Perception scores may suggest general destruction of brain tissue (Golden, 1978).

(5-5) Closed head injuries often produce mild diffuse damage which may demonstrate no gross or severe signs and no effect on Full Scale IQ or on the difference between VIQ and PIQ. With this type of pathology one may also see mixed signs or different levels of impairment because of the contrecoup and shear/strain effect.

(5-6) Infections, general cerebral arteriosclerosis, and degenerative processes which result in atrophy yield generalized deficits (Golden, 1978).

(5-7) Chronic alcoholics often show diffuse impairment with some prominent focal signs in areas such as memory (Golden, 1978).

LATERALIZING SIGNS

The most powerful signs of lateralized lesions are those which indicate differences in performance on the different sides of the body and symptoms of aphasia. The former are seen on the Sensory Perceptual Examination and on the various tests of motor performance while the latter are found on the Aphasia Screening Test. Other possible indicators of lateralization, such as the difference between Verbal and Performance IQ, the difference between scores on the Seashore Rhythm Test and the Speech-sounds Perception Test, and the difference between scores on Parts A and B on the Trail Making Test, are not as powerful indicators of lateralization and should be interpreted much more cautiously (e.g., only when confirming data are established on the sensory and motor tests).

(5-8) When Performance IQ is 20 or more points lower than Verbal IQ on the WAIS, possible right cerebral hemisphere damage is suggested. When the reverse is true, left cerebral hemisphere damage is suspected. One must temper this finding with the fact that the Performance IQ is more likely to be affected by a cerebral lesion than is Verbal IQ due to the fact that the Performance subtests involve new and unique learning, while Verbal subtests measure accumulated knowledge which is least affected by brain damage.

(5-9) A score on Trails B which is substantially poorer than the score on Trails A suggests left hemisphere damage, while a lower score on Part A suggests right cerebral hemisphere damage. This is a weak hypothesis unless substantiated by other data. (Reitan, 1959).

(5-10) Differences in the performance of the two hands on trials one and two on the TPT which exceed the expectations described in Chapter 2 are strong lateralizing signs.

(5-11) Reversal of the TPT relationship becomes more common and, therefore, less significant with increase of age, because transfer of information across the corpus collosum deteriorates and fatigue becomes a more important factor.

(5-12) Differences between the two hands on Finger Oscillation speed and Strength of Grip which exceed the 10% expectation as described in Chapter 2 are strong lateralizing signs.

(5-13) A very poor performance on the Speech-sounds Perception Test in relation to the Seashore Rhythm Test may suggest left hemisphere damage. The reverse may suggest right hemisphere damage, although these are weak signs and should never be interpreted by themselves.

(5-14) Dysnomia, dyslexia, dysgraphia, spelling dyspraxia, dyscalculia, and right-left confusion, in order of significance, suggest left hemisphere damage. Constructional dyspraxia usually suggests right hemisphere damage. It is important to recognize, however, that 15-20% of patients who show constructional dyspraxia have left cerebral hemisphere damage only. This is, therefore, a relatively weak lateralizing sign (Reitan, 1959).

(5-15) Visual suppressions suggest occipital lobe damage in the contralateral hemisphere.

(5-16) Auditory suppressions suggest damage in the contralateral temporal lobe (Reitan, 1959).

(5-17) Extracerebral tumors rarely show lateralization effects on the WAIS (Performance versus Verbal IQ).

(5-18) Localizing or lateralizing signs in the *absence* of depressed FSIQ and with little PIQ-VIQ difference suggest the *absence* of intracerebral tumor or vascular disorder, because these disorders often cause more general damage and lower Performance IQ scores.

(5-19) A subdural hematoma sometimes shows widespread damage, mostly lateralized to the damaged cerebral hemisphere.

(5-20) Tumors and cerebrovascular accidents (CVA) generally result in clear-cut lateralizing signs, although the latter will sometimes be superimposed on a diffuse picture due to a general arteriosclerosis which existed prior to the CVA.

(5-21) A lack of lateralizing signs in the records of schizophrenics may sometimes aid in differentiating them from some brain-damaged patients.

RIGHT HEMISPHERE

In addition to indications of lateralization to the right cerebral hemisphere mentioned in the immediately preceding section, the following hypotheses refer specifically to the right hemisphere:

(5-22) A Block Design score significantly lower than the Picture Arrangement score suggests right parietal-occipital lesions, while a Picture Arrangement score lower than the Block Design score suggests right anterior temporal lesions (Reitan, 1959).

(5-23) If Picture Arrangement and Block Design scores are both depressed, a right temporal-parietal lesion is suggested (Reitan, 1959).

(5-24) If constructional dyspraxia is evident and Block Design is much lower than Picture Arrangement, a right parietal lesion is suggested.

(5-25) Ignoring the left side of a stimulus, as in responding "6-2" to the stimulus 7 SIX 2, suggests a right parietal lesion. This appears to occur most frequently with patients having destructive lesions such as CVAs or intracerebral neoplasms.

LEFT HEMISPHERE

Left hemisphere lesions may be more obvious than right hemisphere lesions on testing because of the importance of the left hemisphere for language functions. The following hypotheses refer specifically to the left hemisphere:

(5-26) A very low score on Similarities suggests left temporal lobe damage. A normal Similarities score, however, does not suggest the absence of left temporal lobe damage. (Reitan, 1959).

(5-27) If aphasic signs are present and Speech-sounds Perception and Seashore Rhythm scores are depressed, a left temporal lesion may be suspected.

(5-28) Aphasic signs are among the strongest indicators of left cerebral hemisphere damage (Reitan, 1959).

(5-29) An attempt to draw the clock instead of writing the word for it as instructed may be a sign of left hemisphere damage.

(5-30) If a patient with an adequate education *adds* 85 and 27 instead of subtracting, damage to the left cerebral hemisphere may be indicated.

(5-31) Most patients read the stimulus 7 SIX 2 as "7-6-2." When a patient reads it as "7-S-I-X-2," left hemisphere damage is suggested.

(5-32) In relatively young adult patients with otherwise healthy brains, impaired language functions (due to recent trauma) appear to improve rapidly; therefore, absence of aphasic symptoms in a young patient with a closed head injury does not rule out trauma to the left side of the head.

LOCALIZING SIGNS

In attempting to localize a lesion it is common to consider first whether the lesion is located more anteriorly or more posteriorly. Since the motor strip is anterior to the fissure of Rolando and the sensory strip is posterior to it, the relative degree of impairment of motor and sensory functions has implications for anterior or posterior location of a lesion. The following hypotheses are relevant to this question:

(5-33) If motor performance on Finger Oscillation and Strength of Grip is depressed, one would expect a lesion in the anterior part of the brain near the motor strip.

(5-34) If TPT performance is more impaired than Finger Oscillation performance with the same hand, a posterior lesion is suggested, i.e., at some distance from the motor strip. If Finger Oscillation is more impaired than TPT with the same hand, a lesion in the anterior part of the contralateral hemisphere is suspected (Reitan, 1959).

(5-35) If TPT scores are depressed and Finger Oscillation is within normal limits, sensory strip involvement is suggested (Reitan, 1959).

(5-36) When there are definite indications of left cerebral hemisphere damage such as dysphasia and lowered Verbal IQ but no indication of left cerebral hemisphere signs on TPT and Finger Oscillation, a focal lesion located at some distance from the motor strip is suggested.

One should next examine the data to see whether still more specific localization to one of the lobes of the cerebral hemisphere is indicated.

FRONTAL LOBES

Lesions of the frontal lobes, especially if they are at some distance anterior to the motor strip, in the prefrontal area, are among the most difficult to identify with the Halstead-Reitan Battery. Emotional reactions are common and impairment of higher level functions such as those seen on the Category Test are often seen; however, one must recognize that the Category Test is sensitive to damage to any part of the brain. Right frontal lobe lesions may be particularly "silent" on the results of the Halstead-Reitan Battery. One patient was seen with a verified right frontal lobe lesion whose only demonstrable deficit on the Battery was an exceptionally low score on the Picture Arrangement subtest of the WAIS. Lezak (1983) has also reported a similar case.

(5-37) If scores on both Category and Part B of Trail Making are below expectation, while other tests are near normal, a focal and static lesion of one or both anterior frontal lobes may be suggested (Reitan, 1959).

(5-38) Expressive dyspraxia signs, dysnomia, spelling apraxia, and dysgraphia suggest left posterior frontal damage (Reitan, 1959).

TEMPORAL LOBES

Temporal lobe lesions may show a number of complex patterns of deficit. Auditory deficits of various kinds are common. If dysphasic signs are seen on the Aphasia Screening Test, it may be useful to examine these further to determine whether the deficits are primarily receptive or expressive. Receptive deficits are more common with temporal lobe involvement. Visual field defects may also result from some temporal lobe lesions and if the hippocampal area is involved, memory impairment may be present. In order to assess memory deficits, a more thorough evaluation of memory should be added to the battery, such as the one suggested by Russell (1975).

(5-39) A very low score on Similarities suggests left temporal lobe damage. A normal Similarities score, however, does not suggest the absence of left temporal lobe damage. (Reitan, 1959).

(5-40) A Block Design score significantly lower than the Picture Arrangement score suggests (right) parietal-occipital lesions, while a Picture Arrangement score lower than the Block Design score suggests (right) anterior temporal lesions (Reitan, 1959).

(5-41) If Picture Arrangement and Block Design scores are both depressed, a right temporal-parietal lesion is suggested (Reitan, 1959).

(5-42) If aphasic signs are present and Speech-sounds Perception and Seashore Rhythm scores are depressed, a left temporal lesion may be suspected.

(5-43) Receptive aphasic signs, visual form agnosia, visual letter agnosia, dyslexia, auditory verbal agnosia, and auditory number agnosia suggest left posterior temporal damage (Reitan, 1959).

(5-44) Visual field defects suggest parietal or temporal lobe damage, often from an intracerebral neoplasm. (Refer to the illustrations in the Appendix for more precise implications of specific field defects.)

(5-45) Auditory suppressions suggest a possibility of damage in the contralateral temporal lobe (Reitan, 1959).

PARIETAL LOBES

Parietal lobe lesions are most commonly reflected in tactile perceptual deficits. They may also affect motor performance on tasks in which effective sensory feedback is necessary for completion of the task. Right parietal lobe lesions may be reflected by difficulty in design copying tasks (constructional dyspraxia), although such deficits are sometimes seen with lesions in the left hemisphere as well. Lack of response to the left half of a stimulus figure is one of the stronger indications of right parietal lobe impairment.

(5-46) A Block Design score significantly lower than the Picture Arrangement score suggests (right) parietal-occipital lesions; a Picture Arrangement score lower than the Block Design score suggests (right) anterior temporal lesions (Reitan, 1959).

(5-47) If Picture Arrangement and Block Design scores are both depressed, a right temporal-parietal lesion is suggested (Reitan, 1959).

(5-48) If constructional dyspraxia is evident and Block Design is much lower than Picture Arrangement, a right parietal lesion is suggested.

(5-49) Ignoring the left side of a stimulus, as in responding "6-2" to the stimulus 7 SIX 2, suggests a right parietal lesion. This appears to occur most frequently with patients having destructive lesions such as CVAs or intracerebral neoplasms.

(5-50) Visual field defects suggest parietal or temporal lobe damage, often from an intracerebral neoplasm. (See Appendix for more precise implications of specific field defects.)

(5-51) Tactile perception is related primarily to parietal lobe functioning; poor scores on fingertip number writing, finger agnosia, tactile coin recognition, and tactual form recognition suggest parietal lesions.

OCCIPITAL LOBES

(5-52) A Block Design score significantly lower than the Picture Arrangement score suggests (right) parietal-occipital lesions; a Picture Arrangement score lower than the Block Design score suggests (right) anterior temporal lesions (Reitan, 1959).

(5-53) Visual suppressions may suggest damage in the contra-lateral hemisphere.

Chapter 6

PROCESS HYPOTHESES

This section includes hypotheses regarding severity, velocity (whether a lesion is static or progressive), prognosis for recovery, and the effects of hospitalization on performance.

SEVERITY

In determining the degree of severity one should consider the general level of performance indicated by the Impairment Index and the scaled scores for those tests recorded on the profile sheet as shown in Chapter 3. These judgments must, however, be tempered by certain other factors which are indicated in the following hypotheses:

(6-1) The significance of an elevated Impairment Index decreases with age after age 45-50.

(6-2) In a brain-damaged person with a high level of education, a low IQ score suggests that the impairment is severe.

(6-3) IQ tends to be negatively correlated with Category scores (Cullum, Steinman, & Bigler, 1984).

(6-4) The Information and Vocabulary subtests from the WAIS are less susceptible to brain damage; therefore, they may offer an indication of premorbid functioning (Golden, 1978).

(6-5) Reversal of TPT relationships becomes more common and less significant with increasing age, because fatigue becomes a more important factor.

(6-6) Misidentification of the circle on tactile form recognition is the most serious error on that test.

If the patient under consideration has been hospitalized for a significant time, the hypotheses in the section on Effects of Hospitalization should also be considered in judging severity.

VELOCITY

In determining whether a lesion is static or progressive, and in determining the speed of progression, the following hypotheses should be considered:

> **(6-7)** If there is a strong indication of brain damage yet IQ scores are relatively unimpaired, a static lesion is suggested.

> **(6-8)** No significant difference between Verbal and Performance IQ suggests diffuse damage and/or a static lesion (Reitan, 1959).

> **(6-9)** If scores on both Category and Part B of Trail Making are below expectation while other tests are near normal, a focal and static lesion of one or both anterior frontal lobes may be suggested (Reitan, 1959).

> **(6-10)** Intact scores on the Speech-sounds Perception Test and the Seashore Rhythm Test indicate that there probably is *not* a rapidly progressive lesion. These scores are good measures of recovery following a CVA or trauma.

This last hypothesis appears to be a particularly important one since patients with rapidly progressive, destructive lesions almost always have severe impairment of attention and concentration which makes adequate performance on these two tests impossible. It should be noted, though, that the converse of this hypothesis is not necessarily true. That is, a very poor performance on these tests does not always imply a rapidly progressive lesion, since many factors may impair performance on these tests which, as indicated in Chapter 2, have complex requirements for successful performance. Careful observation of the precise nature of the patient's performance should aid in identifying the type of deficit that causes the impairment in individual cases.

RECOVERY AND PROGNOSIS

Knowledge of the nature and time of occurrence of a lesion suggests certain hypotheses for recovery and prognosis. For example, there is a commonly seen recovery curve following head injuries which shows a gradual improvement of functioning which may take up to two years post coma to reach maximum spontaneous recovery. The time interval between the injury and the testing, then, has implications for prognosis. The following hypotheses regarding test data also have implications for recovery and prognosis:

(6-11) Prognosis for recovery of language functions is relatively good even with clearcut indications of left cerebral hemisphere damage if the Impairment Index is relatively low and certain other scores such as Category, Speech-sounds Perception, and Seashore Rhythm are adequate.

(6-12) Intact scores on the Speech-sounds Perception Test and the Seashore Rhythm Test indicate that there probably is *not* a rapidly progressive lesion. These scores are good measures of recovery following a CVA or trauma.

EFFECTS OF HOSPITALIZATION

The overall level of performance of schizophrenics on the battery is generally more impaired than that of non-schizophrenics. At least part of this impairment can probably be attributed to the general effects of hospitalization or institutionalization, and one should expect to see a relatively lower level of performance by most patients who have been hospitalized for a significant period at the time of testing, regardless of the reason for hospitalization. For example, many hospitalized patients show a low score on Digit Span; therefore, this is one of the poorest predictors of brain damage.

Strength of Grip and Finger Oscillation speed usually also decline significantly during lengthy hospitalization, but should do so bilaterally, with no indication of lateralization.

Chapter 7

NEUROPATHOLOGICAL CONDITION
HYPOTHESES

This chapter lists the hypotheses regarding the implications of test data for various neuropathological conditions or lesions. It also includes comments about the epidemiology of various lesions and the expected severity, velocity, and prognosis.

TRAUMA

While there are frequently differences in the effects of closed versus penetrating head injuries, they have many epidemiological factors in common. It is clear that people of any age, sex, or position in society may suffer head injuries, but the incidence among some groups is considerably higher. Adolescents and young adults have a particularly high incidence, and certain occupational groups are also at higher risk of suffering head injuries.

The severity of impairment following brain trauma can vary from mild to extremely severe. Patients with gunshot wounds to the head from a close range can show very mild impairment on the Halstead-Reitan Battery. On the other hand, it is not uncommon to see patients who have suffered closed head injuries in automobile accidents which did not result in any penetration of the skull, but who showed severe cognitive and behavioral impairment on these tests. The reverse may also be true, of course, since there are people who show severe impairment following penetrating head injuries and some who show only mild impairment following closed head injuries.

There may be progressive deterioration immediately following traumatic head injury if there is significant uncontrolled bleeding or infection due to penetration by a missile. If the patient survives, there is an expected course of some degree of spontaneous recovery of function over the course of the following 18 to 24 months. For the most part only minor improvement takes place after this natural recovery process.

The prognosis following head injury is determined largely by the severity of the trauma and to some extent by the location of the lesion and the resulting deficits in functioning. For example, a person with a relatively mild trauma that results in a circumscribed lesion may have a very poor prognosis for returning to his/her former activities if functions that were critical for the performance of those activities are impaired.

If a patient has recently suffered a significant head injury, this information will usually be available and the referral question will often be one regarding prognosis and implications for rehabilitation rather than diagnosis. In cases of more remote trauma, this information may not be available and diagnostic questions may be more important. In these cases, epidemiological factors may be helpful. For example, a young adult engaged in a hazardous occupation who shows a pattern of diffuse impairment may be suspected of having an old head injury.

Since severity may be so variable in cases of trauma, it has little implication for diagnosis except in cases of selective degree of severity as indicated below:

> **(7-1)** Static velocity is consistent with a closed head injury, particularly when it occurred some time prior to testing.

> **(7-2)** Closed head injuries may produce mild diffuse damage which may reveal no gross or severe signs and often does not affect Full Scale IQ or differences between VIQ and PIQ. With this type of pathology one may see mixed signs or different levels of impairment because of the contrecoup and shear/strain effects.

> **(7-3)** The Impairment Index tends to be higher in cases with tissue destruction such as intracerebral neoplasms, CVAs, and penetrating head injuries and may be lower in cases of extracerebral neoplasms and some closed head injuries (Golden, 1978).

> **(7-4)** If Finger Oscillation scores are vastly different (example: dominant-3, nondominant-49), a cerebrovascular accident or penetrating head injury is suggested. A closed head injury or tumor can probably be ruled out due to the fact that it would have done more damage to the other cerebral hemisphere.

NEOPLASMS

The epidemiologic factor that is most significant in neoplasms is age. Sex differences are not generally important and other social factors are usually insignificant. Extracerebral neoplasms are the most variable in terms of incidence, occurring more frequently in young people. One should suspect metastases to the brain when there is a picture of spotty impairment shown on the battery in a middle age or older person with a history of a primary carcinoma elsewhere in the body.

As will be seen in the hypotheses below, severity of impairment shown by patients with neoplasms varies considerably, and the degree of severity and the patterning of severity has implications for distinguishing one type of neoplasm from another. Neoplasms, by their very nature, are progressive lesions although the speed of progression may vary considerably. In general, if one suspects the presence of a neoplasm, there should be evidence of a progressive lesion in the test results.

The prognosis with neoplasms varies as a function of type, location, and the stage at which they are identified. Outcome with some extracerebral neoplasms is quite good with surgical intervention, while the prognosis involved in some rapidly growing intracerebral, unencapsulated neoplasms is very poor. Even with surgical intervention, radiation, and chemotherapy, death may result in a few months in many such cases.

The following additional hypotheses relate test data to neoplasms:

(7-5) The absence of any suppression suggests the absence of an acute destructive lesion in the posterior part of the cerebral hemisphere (Reitan, 1959).

(7-6) Extracerebral tumors rarely show lateralization effects on the WAIS (Performance versus Verbal IQ).

(7-7) Extreme sparing of some functions suggests the possibility of an extracerebral neoplasm rather than an intracerebral neoplasm. An example of this would be retention of simple motor speed (tapping) in the presence of other severe deficits.

(7-8) The Impairment Index tends to be higher in cases with tissue destruction such as intracerebral neoplasms, CVAs, and penetrating head injuries, and may be lower in cases of extracerebral neoplasms and mild to moderate closed head injuries (Golden, 1978).

(7-9) Localizing or lateralization signs in the *absence* of depressed FSIQ and with little PIQ-VIQ difference suggest the *absence* of intracerebral tumor or vascular disorder, because such disorders cause more global damage and generally lower Performance IQ.

(7-10) Adequate performance on the Category Test even in the presence of a high Impairment Index and poor performance on other tests does not appear consistent with either intracerebral tumors or massive CVAs, since damage of this type usually impairs abstraction ability, regardless of the location of the lesion.

(7-11) Severe motor and sensory perceptual loss on one side may be associated with either a rapidly progressive intracerebral neoplasm or a severe cerebrovascular problem, but are probably more common to vascular lesions.

(7-12) If Finger Oscillation scores are vastly different (example: dominant-3, nondominant-49), a cerebrovascular accident is suggested. A head injury or tumor can probably be ruled out due to the fact that it would have done more damage to the other cerebral hemisphere.

(7-13) Ignoring the left side of a stimulus, as in responding "6-2" to the stimulus 7 SIX 2, suggests a right parietal lesion. This appears to occur most frequently with patients having destructive lesions such as CVAs or intracerebral neoplasms.

(7-14) A lesion near the optic chiasm may result in one blind eye and one eye with a half field loss. This is sometimes seen in cases with pituitary tumors.

(7-15) Metastatic carcinomas generally show multiple localizing signs plus *very poor* overall performance. For example, if the nonpreferred hand is much poorer than the preferred hand on TPT, time with both hands should be low also. That is, the poor functioning of the nonpreferred hand should interfere with the functioning of the preferred hand. If it does not, the absence of an intracerebral neoplasm, particularly metastatic carcinoma, is suggested (Golden, 1978).

VASCULAR DISORDERS

Vascular disorders encompass a wide range of lesions. They include both congenital and acquired lesions which may exhibit the full range of severity, velocity, and prognosis. The most commonly encountered and most significant types are cerebrovascular accidents (CVAs) and cerebral arteriosclerosis.

While the less common types of vascular lesions (e.g., congenital vascular anomalies) are obviously seen in patients of all ages, CVAs and cerebral arteriosclerosis occur most often in later life. The incidence is greater among males than females, although this sex difference is decreasing. Histories of hypertension, smoking, and heavy use of alcohol are associated with a higher incidence of certain vascular disorders. Of special note is the fact that an increased incidence of CVAs has been noted among younger women who have used oral contraceptives for a period of time. Consequently, if one sees a pattern of test results that suggests the possibility of a CVA in a woman in her 20s or 30s, at which age a CVA would not ordinarily be expected, inquiry should be made about the use of such medications.

The severity of impairment resulting from congenital vascular disorders is generally mild, whereas CVAs may result in significant impairment. Cerebral arteriosclerotic disease may cause either mild, moderate, or severe impairment at any point in time. The severity of impairment of such functions as orientation and memory may vary, even daily, in some cases of arteriosclerosis, perhaps due to transient ischemic attacks (TIAs).

The prognosis following a CVA depends on the size and location of the damage and the functions that are impaired as a direct result, as well as the role that these functions have previously played in the patient's life. It is important to note that people who have had a CVA have a higher probability of subsequent occurrence than those who have never experienced such trauma. The prognosis for people with cerebral arteriosclerosis must be considered generally poor, since this is a progressive, degenerative disorder for which there is no effective treatment.

A history of previous vascular disorders, including but not limited to cerebral vascular disorders, predisposes one toward a CVA; therefore, such a history may aid in distinguishing between a CVA and other lesions which show a similar pattern of test results. This also means that the sharply localized pattern of test results characteristic of a CVA may sometimes be superimposed on a diffuse pattern characteristic of cerebral arteriosclerosis.

(7-16) Localizing or lateralizing signs in the *absence* of depressed FSIQ and with little PIQ-VIQ difference suggest the *absence* of intracerebral tumor or vascular disorder, because these disorders cause more global damage and generally lower performance IQs.

(7-17) Adequate performance on the Category Test, even in the presence of a high Impairment Index and poor performance on other tests, does not appear consistent with either intracerebral tumors or massive CVAs since damage of this type usually impairs abstraction ability regardless of the location of the lesion.

(7-18) Severe motor and sensory perceptual loss on one side may be associated with either a rapidly progressive intracerebral neoplasm or a severe cerebrovascular problem, but is probably more common with vascular lesions.

(7-19) If Finger Oscillation scores are vastly different (example: dominant-3, nondominant-49), a CVA is suggested. A head injury or tumor can probably be ruled out due to the fact that it would have done more damage to the other cerebral hemisphere.

(7-20) Ignoring the left side of a stimulus, as in responding "6-2" to the stimulus 7 SIX 2, suggests a right parietal lesion. This appears to occur most frequently with patients having destructive lesions such as CVAs or intracerebral neoplasms.

DEGENERATIVE DISEASES

The disorders discussed here all result from a gradual deterioration of tissue in one or more parts of the brain. While some of them have several features in common, the striking differences require that they be considered separately.

Cortical Atrophy (Primary Degenerative Dementia)

Diseases such as Alzheimer's and Pick's result in a general diffuse atrophy of the cortex. They are distinguished by histological differences, but neuropsychologically they are indistinguishable from each other. They occur commonly in people in their 60s and above, but sometimes occur in patients in their 50s as well.

The severity of impairment ranges from mild to very severe. Most cases seen for neuropsychological assessment will show at least moderate severity, and most severely impaired patients will be virtually untestable with many of the assessment procedures in the Halstead-Reitan Battery. This results from their extreme impairment of concentration and attention and their inability to follow complex instructions.

These disorders are progressive and the rate of progression may range from relatively slow to fairly rapid. Definite evidence of deterioration can usually be seen on retesting after a year. Since there is no effective treatment, prognosis must always be considered poor. The most important questions for the neuropsychologist are usually the ones related to how much self-care these people are capable of, and how structured and protected their living situation needs to be at any point in time. Most of them will eventually require skilled nursing care, but through identification of strengths and weaknesses, one may be able to avoid premature institutionalization. This is important since overly protective and restrictive environments will almost always result in regression and more rapid deterioration of functioning. The identification by the neuropsychologist of strengths and weaknesses and their implications for daily functioning is important to help other clinicians and family members understand the optimal amount of care that these patients need.

Patients with cortical atrophy often show considerable confusion during testing. This may be manifested by difficulty in understanding even simple instructions and an apparent disorientation even in a relatively familiar environment. Global impairment will be present on neuropsychological examination.

Hydrocephalus

Hydrocephalus occurs most often in infants; when it does, there is little question about the diagnosis due to the obvious gross physical deformity of the head. It occurs more rarely in adults and is not obvious since the bones of the skull have fused, preventing the enlargement of the cranium seen in infants.

Behavioral effects are generally severe, and the disorder is progressive with a grim prognosis without surgical intervention. Installation of a shunt to reduce cerebrospinal fluid pressure produces good results in many cases.

If the neuropsychologist sees a pattern of diffuse, progressive impairment in a child or younger adult, the possibility of hydrocephalus should be considered. Such cases should be referred for neurological or neurosurgical evaluation since lumbar puncture, pneumoencephalograms, and CAT scans can provide a definite diagnosis and surgical intervention can be considered.

Chronic Alcoholism

Those alcoholics seen for neuropsychological evaluation are most frequently chronic abusers in their 40s and older. Alcoholism is becoming a more serious problem at an earlier age, though, and increasing numbers of younger patients will be seen in the future. The incidence of alcoholism among women also appears to be increasing, or at least recognized more often. It generally takes a number of years of heavy drinking to produce neuropsychological deficits, and it is this history that is significant regardless of the age of the person.

The severity of deficits may range from mild to severe and the degree of severity appears related to factors such as duration and quantity of consumption, as well as constitutional factors. If the person continues to drink heavily, the deterioration will be gradually progressive. With abstinence there will be some degree of improvement in some areas, but in many cases there will remain a static profile of impairment following this acute recovery period. The prognosis is determined by severity of impairment, presence or absence of abstinence, and constitutional factors.

> **(7-21)** Alcoholics do most poorly on the Category Test and often exhibit poor scores on the entire test battery.
>
> **(7-22)** Memory deficits are commonly seen in chronic alcoholics.

Even when performance on the Wechsler Memory Scale is adequate, significant deficits may be demonstrated by using the 30 minute delayed recall procedure designed by Russell (1975). When this procedure is used, the stories which may have been repeated fairly accurately on the initial trial often become woefully distorted on the delayed recall. These distortions can show indications of confabulation, with frequent personal references, even in patients who do not demonstrate clinical evidence of a fully developed Korsakoff's Syndrome.

This pattern of performance may have definite implications for the ability to function independently. Sometimes such patients appear to be capable of independent functioning on the basis of observations of their behavior in an institutional setting, but their impairment of short term memory may cause serious problems if they are living in an independent environment.

Parkinsonism

Parkinson's disease occurs most often among older people, with the incidence progressively increasing with advance in age beyond 50. The severity may range from mild to moderate and occasionally severe. It is generally a slowly progressive disorder and the pattern seen on the results of the battery is usually a relatively static one. The prognosis is generally poor, although medical treatment or even surgical intervention may be helpful in some cases. The most obvious symptoms are cerebellar tremor and gait disturbance. Motor problems are a common feature of this disorder and they may frequently be seen as a resting tremor. Micrographia is sometimes seen in patients with Parkinsonism and may be noted when the person is required to write various words and sentences on the Aphasia Screening Test or when drawing the cross and key.

> **(7-23)** Patients with Parkinson's disease often perform poorly on the Category Test, tend to have relatively high impairment indices, and perform poorly on Trail Making and motor tests; their IQs may be in the average range. (Reitan & Boll, 1971)

Multiple Sclerosis

Multiple sclerosis (MS) is a degenerative disease in which demyelination occurs at numerous locations within the central nervous system including, in some cases, both the brain and the spinal cord. This results in a wide variety of neurological symptoms. The earliest symptoms usually occur in the 20s and 30s and may go into remission for many years. This disorder, consequently, is elusive and sometimes overlooked or misdiagnosed until a different symptom of impairment in another area of the central nervous system occurs, which may be 10 or more years later.

This is, then, a slowly progressive disorder with frequent remission. The pattern of test results on the battery is usually a static one which ranges from mild to moderate severity in ambulatory populations, with greater impairment seen in hospitalized patients. The prognosis for continued functioning is fairly good in many cases, although motor or sensory problems may create severe limitations for some people.

Because of the wide dispersion of multiple lesions throughout the central nervous system, the pattern of results on the battery is often a spotty one with sharp areas of deficits concomitant with many well preserved functions. For example, one may see greater impairment of motor functions on one side of the body with greater impairment of sensory functions on the opposite side of the body.

Since cases with multiple metastatic carcinomas also often exhibit spotty patterns of impairment, it is important to differentiate between these two disorders. This is usually not difficult since metastatic carcinomas result in more severe impairment and show evidence of a rapidly progressive disorder. In such cases, for example, scores on the Seashore Rhythm Test would probably be very poor.

(7-24) Patients with multiple sclerosis will often show both weakness and poor sensory perceptual performance.

(7-25) IQ is usually not affected in cases of MS (except in some cases when motor deficits interfere with Performance IQ) and "higher order" functions are generally well preserved.

If the neuropsychologist suspects the presence of previously undiagnosed MS on the basis of test results, inquiry should be made about *past* neurological symptoms even when they are currently not present. This should include constant or transient:

- Visual problems such as transient blindness or a loss of acuity.

- Auditory deficits.

- Tactile sensation impairment such as tingling and numbness.

- Weakness in any part of the body.

- Balance, coordination, or gait problems.

- Bladder difficulties including urgency, incontinence, or retention.

As noted in Chapter 1, a measure of CFF may also be a useful neuropsychological test to aid in identifying MS. Daley, Swank, and Ellison (1979), Fishbach, Harrer, and Wagner (1973), Jarvis and Buchholz (1981), Parsons and Miller (1957), and Titcombe and Willison (1961) have demonstrated useful and similar hit rates for this purpose. Of these studies, however, only the one by Jarvis and Buchholz appears to have utilized procedures and developed norms that have potential clinical utility.

Chapter 8

THE NEUROPSYCHOLOGICAL INTERVIEW

In much of the neuropsychological literature one may get the impression that the neuropsychologist never sees the patients. The patients instead are examined by technicians and the neuropsychologist only studies data generated by the technician's examination of the patient. This has, in fact, been the procedure for many neuropsychologists operating in research settings. When validation studies of neuropsychological batteries have been conducted, the neuropsychologist has typically performed blind analyses of the data (Reitan, 1975). One of the best ways for the beginning neuropsychologist to develop a thorough understanding of brain-behavior relationships and to begin to formulate diagnostic statements is through the sole study of neuropsychological test data. This is the approach used in Chapter 11 of this Guide.

On the other hand, the practicing clinical neuropsychologist should be concerned with far more than simply this type of academic or research exercise. In those cases where he or she is called on to assist in formulating a diagnosis, the neuropsychologist should use all of the available information and not rely solely on test data. Furthermore, the neuropsychologist is often called on to do far more than simply arrive at a neurodiagnosis. As pointed out in Chapter 3, the most important contribution of the neuropsychologist is one of identifying the cognitive and behavioral correlates and prognosis of a known lesion, and using this information in the formulation of a rehabilitation plan. For these purposes, an understanding of the approaches to neuropsychological interviewing described here are essential.

The question arises of how the neuropsychological interview is different from a clinical interview performed by a clinical psychologist or psychiatrist, a social history or social systems interview performed by either a social worker or other clinician, and a neurological history or interview performed by a neurologist. The clinical psychologist or psychiatrist will usually be primarily concerned with psychological factors such as the patient's mental status, intellectual functioning, mood, affect, thinking and perceptual processes. The more socially oriented clinician will focus on social systems factors such as interpersonal relationships, family and work history, and other related social issues. The neurologist will be primarily interested in a history of physical illnesses and conditions which may suggest neurologically impairing events.

The most common approach to integrating the data from all of these perspectives is for each of the experts to gather data independently from interviews and other sources and to come together in a team case conference in which a diagnosis is developed and a treatment or rehabilitation plan is formulated. The advantage to this approach is that each of these clinical specialists has certain expertise and a unique sensitivity to problems in his or her own area of specialization. The disadvantage, however, is that each specialist may tend to assume that the disorder presented by the patient can be explained by factors that he or she uncovers. The subtle ways in which physical, psychological, and social factors interact may not be fully appreciated and the resulting formulation and plan may consequently be less than optimal.

An alternative approach is to conduct an integrated neuropsychological interview in which the interaction of these factors is studied and assessed. This focus on the interaction of various factors is what may make the neuropsychological interview particularly valuable. The disadvantage to this approach is that any single clinician, including the neuropsychologist, may lack knowledge and skill in one or more of these specialized areas. It is necessary in most cases, therefore, for each of the clinical specialists to conduct independent investigations and to contribute to the total formulation and plan. If the neuropsychologist, however, is aware of the variety of factors which can influence the patient's behavior and the interactions among these factors, he or she can enhance the total team effort and play a major role in generating the most useful formulation and plan.

This requires a recognition that a brain-impairing event, for example, may lead to a complex interaction of neurological, psychological, and social factors which determine the ultimate symptomatic behavior that is seen. Such an event sets off a chain of other events that all contribute to the eventual clinical picture. This chain of events may be thought of as occurring in a sequence like the following: 1) A lesion in the central nervous system occurs. The patient's behavior is influenced by the physical factors of the nature, location, and velocity of the lesion and the developmental stage of the organism at the time of the occurrence of the lesion. 2) This produces some immediate impairment of functions such as sensory or memory deficits. 3) The patient has some awareness of the change or impairment of function. The degree of awareness depends on factors such as intelligence, education, and environmental (including social) demands on the patient. 4) The patient then reacts to this awareness that "something is wrong" and to the reaction of other people in the environment. This reaction depends on such factors as premorbid personality and intelligence, among others. For example, a patient with a history of low self-esteem may react by feeling inadequate, worthless, and depressed. On the other hand, given a different premorbid personality and/or involvement with a different social system that has different expectations of the patient, the patient may project the blame for the changes in functioning onto others and appear quite paranoid.

Some examples may clarify this process. A 55-year-old male was brought to a mental health center appearing severely paranoid with extensive delusions of persecution by the Mafia. When seen at the mental health center, these delusions were quite pervasive, affecting most spheres of his life and resulting in his taking elaborate steps to protect himself from the assaults that he anticipated. Closer inquiry revealed that his fears had manifested themselves initially at night. He had become anxious on going to bed with the lights out, and it seemed that he had been afraid of the dark, although he quickly projected these fears onto the environment. A thorough history revealed that he had contracted syphilis 30 to 35 years prior to being seen at the mental health center, and physical examination and laboratory studies revealed that he now had tertiary syphilis (tabes dorsalis). As the afferent pathways in the dorsal area of the spinal cord became impaired and he could not walk well in the dark, he became aware of this impairment. His personality was such that he dealt with the awareness by beginning to project the blame for it. As he did this, and as the neurological impairment gradually became more severe, he found further confirmation for his projections in the environment and developed a full blown paranoid system in a process much like that described by Cameron (1959).

In another case, a 30-year-old man was seen with complaints of depression, feelings of inadequacy, and frequent uncontrolled crying spells. In recent months he had been unable to perform adequately in his job. Three months prior to being seen at a mental health center, he had experienced a motorcycle accident in which he suffered a head injury resulting in a right frontal hematoma. The neurosurgeon who had treated him indicated that this appeared to be resolving satisfactorily with no detectable clinical neurological residuals. A neuropsychological interview revealed that this was a man who had had a very deprived childhood and had felt basically inadequate and insecure but had defended against this by assuming a front of a "big tough man." This was reflected, for example, in the nickname that he had adopted for himself, "Hunter." This nickname reflected his interest and active engagement in a number of outdoor activities and sports. The interview further revealed that his problems on the job were a result of inadequate ability to cope with spatial relationships, and it seemed likely that this would also impair his ability to find his way around in the mountains while engaging in the outdoor activities that had been important to him before the accident. When he was no longer able to handle the same job that he had had before or to engage satisfactorily in some of his previous activities, he felt that he had "lost face." He was, therefore, unable to keep up the tough front of the "Hunter." His earlier, long defended against, childhood feelings of inadequacy became apparent to him, resulting in the depression and crying spells. Subsequent neuropsychological testing revealed a mild but definite right cerebral hemisphere deficit which could account for the difficulty in handling spatial relationships and suggested certain changes in his work and other activities. Neither the psychological factors nor the minimal neurological deficits, which could not be detected on physical examination, alone could have explained this clinical picture. A satisfactory explanation required an understanding of the interaction of both. For other examples of the interaction of these factors see Jarvis and Barth (1979) and Jarvis and Vollman (1983).

There are two general types of neuropsychological interview. The type of interview is determined by the question which the neuropsychologist is attempting to answer at a particular point in any case study. The first type is a screening interview, which is used when no definite neurological diagnosis has been made and the need is to determine whether complete neuropsychological evaluation and/or neurological assessment is required. There may be several different types of indications for the screening interview.

First, there may be indications seen in the mental status examination of the patient. These may include signs of disorientation, confusion, memory problems, or communication difficulties which do not clearly appear to be a result of a thought disorder. Various complaints that patients present may also provide an indication for such a screening interview. These may include complaints of poor memory, sensory or motor problems, or any other change in functioning which could be a result of brain damage.

An atypical psychiatric history may also provide a clear indication for a neuropsychological screening interview. For example, a 50-year-old woman was seen in a mental hospital after having been treated by a psychiatrist in the community with large doses of phenothiazine for a diagnosis of schizophrenia. This woman's history was atypical in that neither she nor her family reported any previous history of mental illness prior to the gradual onset of her present problems a few months prior to her admission. Her admission to the hospital was precipitated by an alleged suicide attempt in which she turned on the gas stove in her apartment without lighting the burner. This woman had a history of very good vocational adjustment in the past. She had held a very responsible job for a number of years but about two years prior to admission had apparently begun to function less adequately on the job and had gradually shifted to less responsible jobs and eventually stopped working entirely. The neuropsychological interview revealed that she was somewhat confused and unable to follow even very simple instructions. She left the interview room on the ward at one point to go to her bedroom to get her glasses, and was unable to find her way back to the interview room which was only a few doors away. She revealed deficits in her ability to handle many requirements of independent everyday living. A careful investigation of the alleged suicide attempt seemed to indicate the likelihood of confusion or a failure to remember that the pilot light on her stove was not working. Neuropsychological screening tests were administered, and revealed evidence of deficits in a number of areas, involving both cerebral hemispheres. Subsequently, a complete neuropsychological test battery was administered and the results were interpreted as being consistent with diffuse cortical atrophy. With this information, it was possible to identify the amount of structure that this woman required for placement in a semi-sheltered living situation in the community. It was also possible to counsel the family about the prognosis, which indicated that this woman would probably require a more sheltered situation in the future, since it appeared that she was suffering from a degenerative disease.

Other puzzling diagnostic questions may also provide an indication for a neuropsychological interview. These may include disorders such as the type of unprovoked explosive behavior which has been described by Bach-Y-Rita, Lion, Climent, and Ervin (1971). This type of clinical picture, combined with evidence from neuropsychological interviews regarding possible brain-impairing events, may suggest the need for EEG studies with nasopharyngeal leads to determine the possibility of psychomotor seizure activity resulting from a temporal lobe focus. This may be alleviated subsequently by administration of anticonvulsant medications.

An outline for identifying factors which can produce brain impairment but which might otherwise be overlooked in a standard clinical psychological interview is presented on the following pages. It is important for the interviewer to keep in mind the interaction of factors described earlier, which produce the resulting symptomatic behavior seen following such impairment. The interviewer should inquire not only whether such events occurred, but also how the patient and others perceived them and reacted to them. It is also important to remember that this is an outline for a screening interview only, and such an interview will seldom result in a definitive diagnosis. A combination of positive findings on several of the factors listed here may, however, suggest the need for more complete neuropsychological and/or neurological evaluation.

The neuropsychologist should view this as a guide to important data to be collected, but should not use it as an exhaustive checklist. The neuropsychological interview should be conducted in the same way that any other good clinical interview is, taking account of important factors such as rapport with the patient.

The interviewer should also be very observant of all aspects of the patient's behavior. It is helpful to meet the patient in the waiting room or on the ward. This provides an opportunity to observe the patient's station (the way he or she stands and sits) and gait. If the patient is met by the interviewer on a ward and escorted to an interview room, there may be an opportunity at the end of the interview to assess the patient's ability to find his or her way back to the ward. The interviewer should introduce himself or herself to the patient by name at the beginning of the interview and may then assess the patient's gross attention and memory at a later point by asking whether the patient recalls the interviewer's name.

Other observations should include such factors as any evidence of weakness, particularly on one side of the body in arms, legs, or face. The patient's speech should be assessed, noting particularly articulation problems or any hesitation in choosing the right words. Gross evidence of auditory or visual acuity impairment should be noted. It is often important to ask whether the patient ordinarily wears glasses if he or she does not have them on. Tremors should be noted, including the observations of whether they are resting tremors (evident when the patient is not carrying out some purposeful act) or intention tremors (evident when the patient attempts to carry out some action).

Scars, bruises, or other evidence of injury should be noted and investigated. Even peripheral injuries may have resulted in loss of consciousness and may at times have been accompanied by head injuries which are not presently visible. Recent bruises may be evidence of injuries sustained during convulsions or other episodes of loss of consciousness, or may have resulted from disturbances in balance.

The patient's mood and affect should be assessed with particular note of highly labile affect. If mood disturbances are noted, inquiry should be made about changes in mood and the onset in relationship to other factors.

OUTLINE FOR NEUROPSYCHOLOGICAL HISTORY

The following outline lists a number of important points that should be considered in the neuropsychological history. Included are various neurological symptoms, indications of traumatic events, and deviations from normal developmental patterns. A consideration of all of these factors may provide clues to the presence of brain damage as well as its etiology and prognosis.

Prenatal

1. Illnesses of the mother during pregnancy (e.g., German measles, various chemical addictions).
2. Medications or other drugs taken by the mother during pregnancy.
3. Age of mother at birth of patient (e.g., over 35 years of age).

Labor and Delivery

1. Abnormal length or difficulty of labor (e.g., longer than 8 - 10 hours).
2. Prematurity and birth weight.
3. Forceps delivery.
4. Possible anoxia in the child during delivery.
5. Any deformity of the head at birth which does not resolve spontaneously.

Childhood

1. High fevers.
2. Convulsions.

3. Fainting spells.
4. Childhood illnesses, especially stressing illnesses such as meningitis and encephalitis and any complications of other illnesses.

Early Development

1. Delay in learning to walk.
2. Delay in learning to talk.

Early School Years

1. Difficulty in learning to read.
2. Behavioral problems in school or at home (hyperactivity/hypoactivity).

General

1. Any significant injury, especially to the head.
2. Visual problems.
3. Hearing problems.
4. Other sensory problems such as of touch, taste, smell, etc.
5. Blackouts.
6. Seizures.
7. Any disturbance of consciousness.
8. Use of medications (type, when, how long, reason for taking).
9. Use of alcohol (how extensively, when, for how long).
10. Use of other drugs (type of drugs, how extensively, when, for how long).
11. Memory problems (nature, onset).
12. Language disturbances (failure to recognize words or objects, problems with articulation).
13. Disturbances in coordination and gait.
14. Episodes of uncontrolled behavior in the absence of provocation.

The prenatal period, although sometimes ignored, is important because brain-impairing events during this period may permanently establish the "functional ceiling" of abilities. If deficits are identified while the patient is still a child, they may have implications for remedial training or treatment. Illnesses of the mother during pregnancy, such as rubella, may sometimes produce subtle birth defects that have implications for the future mental health of the child. It is well established that taking certain medications or other drugs during pregnancy can result in similar effects. The incidence of certain birth defects also tends to increase with the increased age of the mother at the time of pregnancy.

The labor and delivery process also provides possibilities for physical trauma. A difficult or abnormal labor may produce anoxia, and other factors may result in the neonate having breathing difficulty immediately following delivery. Trauma may result from the use of forceps and may be indicated by significant deformity of the neonate's head. Substantial prematurity may result in a lag in the development of the central nervous system. An abnormally high birth weight may cause trauma by resulting in a difficult delivery.

Many incidents during childhood that may be overlooked by parents can indicate events that impair nervous system functioning and may be elicited by careful questioning. Unusually high fevers, fainting spells not associated with heat, hyperventilation, asphyxia, or convulsions may be indicative of central nervous system impairment. Childhood illnesses may also have the same effect, especially meningitis, encephalitis, or various complications resulting from other more common childhood illnesses.

Deviations from normal developmental patterns in functions such as walking and talking can suggest central nervous system impairment that may eventually lead to aberrant behavior patterns seen at later evaluation. Similarly, during school years, difficulty in learning to read or write or behavior problems such as hyperactivity or hypoactivity may be indicative of the minimal brain dysfunction syndrome (e.g., Klonoff & Low, 1974) that can pose a complicated picture later when confounded with psychological and social factors.

Regardless of the time of occurrence, any serious head injury may be significant. Sensory problems in any modality should be investigated, because these may be signs of events that can have neurological implications. Also, blackouts may imply altered states of consciousness due to impaired central nervous system functioning.

Various types of medications may be significant in different ways. In some cases, they may indicate chemical abuse problems. In others, they may give clues to problems such as the minimal brain dysfunction syndrome (use of amphetamines) or convulsive disorders (use of anticonvulsant medications or barbiturates). The use of alcohol or other drugs may lead to toxic states which can have long lasting effects on behavior.

While memory problems may be the result of a "functional" disorder unrelated to identifiable brain damage, they may also be among the earliest or most prominent indications of brain-impairing lesions. Similarly, language disturbances may be dysphasic in nature as opposed to being the result of a thought disorder. It may be necessary to assess possible language disturbances with a brief aphasia screening examination such as the Reitan Indiana Aphasia Screening Test in order to distinguish between these two types of disorders.

Disturbances of either coordination or gait may reflect not only the effects of anxiety, but also either peripheral or central nervous system disorder. Significant disturbances in this area should be evaluated by a neurologist to assess the possible etiology.

Finally, episodes of uncontrolled behavior in the absence of provocation may suggest convulsive disorders of the type described by Bach-Y-Rita et al. (1971). These can be compounded by psychological and social factors and may be alleviated by anticonvulsant medications.

The second type of neuropsychological interview is the integrating or clarifying interview. This is called for when the presence of a brain lesion is verified or strongly suspected as a result of a definite history of disease, trauma, positive findings on a neuropsychological assessment or neurological examination, or other physical evaluation procedures. The general considerations described above regarding how the neuropsychological interview should be conducted also apply to the integrating or clarifying interview, although the outline for the history is generally not needed. Instead, the focus of this interview should be the determination of how the immediate deficits resulting from the brain lesion have interacted with other factors. The neuropsychologist should assess the patient's awareness of the functional deficits in areas such as sensation, motor skills, memory, and cognition. The interviewer should attempt to determine how the patient has reacted to this awareness. Determination should also be made of degree of awareness other people in the patient's social environment have of these deficits and how they have reacted to them. This may require additional interviews with family members and others. The interviewer should determine both from the patient interview and other informants how the functional deficits and the person's awareness of them are affecting everyday functioning on the job, at home, and at school. As indicated in Chapter 1, the neuropsychologist may also use this interview as an opportunity to identify the need for further assessment. This may require either additional neuropsychological testing, or additional neurological tests.

Finally, this clarifying interview provides an opportunity to formulate suggestions for more effective coping and rehabilitation and to make an initial presentation of these suggestions to the patient and family. This may be the most important aspect of the evaluation process from the point of view of the patient and family and may help to dispel exaggerated fears regarding the patient's future.

DIFFERENTIAL INDICATIONS FOR NEUROPSYCHOLOGICAL OR NEUROLOGICAL ASSESSMENT

Questions will frequently arise regarding the different indications for neuropsychological or neurological assessment. These questions fall into three general categories: 1) Based on the type of initial interview described in the first part of this chapter, what are the indications for a medical-neurological consultation, as opposed to only a neuropsychological evaluation? 2) Based on the neuropsychological evaluation, what are the indications for a follow-up medical-neurological consultation? 3) What are the general indications for a neuropsychological evaluation in a medical setting?

In the first of these situations, it is imperative that medical consultation be sought immediately in cases where indications of acute neurological problems are found. These include rapid onset of significant motor or sensory problems, severe headache, and delirium. In cases with less severe problems, less rapid onset, and absence of delirium, medical consultation may be delayed until a neuropsychological evaluation is completed. For example, a patient who shows weakness on the right side of the body and aphasic signs with a recent sudden onset may have had a CVA, and an immediate medical consultation should be requested.

In the second type of case, following a neuropsychological evaluation, any case in which the neuropsychological evaluation leads to a suspicion of a treatable neurological disorder should be referred for consultation. This includes all cases of suspected acute or progressive conditions, and chronic or static disorders whose etiology cannot be determined by the history. Wherever there is any doubt, the psychologist should request consultation.

Finally, neuropsychological examinations in medical centers are often requested by psychiatrists, neurologists, and neurosurgeons, in order to help confirm questionable diagnoses and develop a baseline evaluation of behavior and cognition to determine if intervention is successful. Neuropsychological assessment can help to delineate the effects of medication, neurosurgical procedures, and other therapies, as well as chart the recovery process so that practical questions regarding the need for continued hospitalization, daily supervision, return to work and family, and other management/treatment issues can be addressed.

Note. Portions of this chapter are from "The neglect of physical-neurological factors in community mental health practice: A proposal for a better balance," 1979, *Clinical Neuropsychology, 1,* pgs. 20-23. Reprinted by permission.

Chapter 9

THE NEUROLOGICAL EXAMINATION

The neuropsychologist needs to know what his/her neurological colleague does in examining the nervous system. A knowledge of these procedures will contribute to an understanding of how the neurological examination and the neuropsychological examination should be complementary. It will also illustrate the indications for the more specialized neurological-radiological examination techniques described in the next chapter.

The neurological examination may concentrate on areas of suspected problems. At other times it may be a very brief "screening examination." The most superficial of such screening examinations has been described, perhaps facetiously, by one neurologist as consisting of simply an examination of the cranial nerves and testing for the Babinski reflex. On the other hand, the neurological examination may be an extremely thorough and time consuming procedure. The following outline for a "routine" neurological examination is similar to one described by Steegmann (1962) and is typical of the complete neurological examination.

The neurologist usually begins by obtaining a neurological and medical history. Steegman (1962) indicates that a number of points in the neurological history are particularly crucial. The reader will see a marked similarity between these points and the outline for a neuropsychological interview described in Chapter 8.

Changes in state of consciousness are evaluated by the neurologist. These conditions may range from the transitory clouding of consciousness seen in some petit mal seizures to the stupor or coma which may accompany severe lesions of the central nervous system.

Headaches are given special attention, including a review of the quality, location and intensity of the pain, as well as various factors which may aggravate or relieve the pain. Dizziness or vertigo is evaluated with a focus on the

85

factors that produce it and alleviate it, as well as other related sensations and conditions such as nausea and vomiting. Disturbances in pain sensation should be evaluated, with special attention to the nature of the pain, its frequency, duration, location and intensity. Disturbances in pain sensation may also include a decrease in sensations of pain with stimuli which would normally produce painful sensations. Subjective reports of visual disturbances are recorded with attention to such factors as decreased acuity, blurring, or double vision. Similarly, disturbances of smell and taste are evaluated. Any history of convulsions is explored thoroughly with special attention to the presence of auras, loss of consciousness, and the nature and location of motor contractions. A history of vomiting is explored to determine whether it was accompanied by nausea, pain, headache, or abdominal symptoms.

Motor weakness reported by the patient is evaluated to determine features of onset and course, location and duration of the weakness, and the conditions which relieve or exacerbate it. Bladder and bowel problems are explored to determine their specific nature, onset, and relationship to other factors. Difficulties in gait are considered, particularly to determine whether they are related to weakness or lack of coordination. The relationship of gait difficulties to other factors such as darkness may be particularly important. Disturbances of speech are investigated to determine whether they are aphasic in nature or associated with problems in articulation or memory. Related difficulties in chewing and swallowing are also frequently explored in connection with speech disturbances. Sleep patterns are examined to determine the duration of sleep, difficulty in sleeping, or excessive drowsiness. The focus here is often on changes in the sleep pattern. Autonomic functions, including sweating, palpitation and digestive disturbances, are investigated.

A general medical and psychiatric history of both the patient and family members is typically obtained. A family history is particularly important when there is concern about convulsive disorders or hereditary conditions such as Huntington's chorea.

The equipment needed for the routine clinical neurological examination is fairly simple. It usually includes a flashlight, ophthalmoscope, several pins, cotton for testing tactile sensation, a percussion hammer, and tuning fork. Materials for testing sensations of temperature, taste, and smell are often also included.

Many neurologists begin the actual physical examination by testing the cranial nerves. In a superficial examination the olfactory nerve may not be tested. When it is, this is done by asking the patient to identify the odor of substances such as oil of peppermint or ground coffee. The optic nerve is evaluated in several ways. A simple test of visual acuity may be done. The visual fields are mapped roughly by a direct confrontation technique similar to that used in the Sensory Perceptual Examination of the Halstead-Reitan Battery. If this leads to suspicion of visual field defects, more sophisticated techniques may be employed by the neurologist or by an ophthalmologist. Finally, the optic fundi are examined with an ophthalmoscope.

The third, fourth, and sixth cranial nerves are functionally related and examined together. This consists of an examination of the external eyes and their positions, the pupils, and certain pupillary reflexes and eye movements under various conditions. The fifth cranial nerve is examined in both its motor and sensory divisions. In the former, for example, mouth and jaw movements are evaluated; in the latter, sensations of various parts of the face are tested. The seventh cranial nerve is evaluated by having the patient perform various motor acts such as frowning, closing the eyes tightly, or elevating the eyebrows. Taste sensation may also be tested using four basic substances: sweet, sour, bitter, and salt.

The most common testing of the eighth nerve is a fairly crude test of auditory acuity. If decreased acuity is noted, further testing with a tuning fork may be done to determine whether the decrease in acuity is of a conduction deficit or nerve deficit type. More definitive evaluation of hearing loss requires a specialized audiometric examination. The ninth and tenth nerves are evaluated by observing the position and movement of the palate and tongue. The eleventh nerve is tested by having the patient move his/her shoulders up toward the ears against resistance to the examiner's hands on the patient's shoulders, and by having the patient turn his/her head to one side against resistance to the examiner's attempt to pull the chin back. The twelfth cranial nerve is evaluated by examination of the position and movement of the patient's tongue and by having the patient repeat certain words or phrases which require complex tongue movement and coordination. At some point in the neurological examination, the neurologist typically evaluates the size and shape of the head, skull tenderness or pain, and sometimes sounds heard on percussion of the skull.

The extent of the examination of the patient's motor system will vary considerably from one examination to another, depending on the nature of the patient's complaint and the observations made in the first general portions of this examination. These include a general inspection of the patient's ability to carry out certain simple motor tasks such as walking in various manners, bending his/her body in various directions, and squatting. The other general evaluation of the motor system includes an assessment of the patient's station and gait. The term station refers to the way in which a person stands, and the term gait refers to the way in which he or she walks. General muscle tone, muscle movement, and muscle strength are evaluated. When specific problems are suspected, assessment of muscle strength is very thorough and complex, including testing of many different muscle groups. Grading of muscle strength is typically done by the neurologist on a relatively crude six point

scale. More refined testing of muscle strength requires utilization of the specialized techniques of electromyography.

When most people think of a neurological examination, they probably
think of the testing of reflexes. This is because the examination of reflexes is
done more frequently than some other parts of the neurological examination.
Both deep reflexes, which are produced by stimulation of a tendon or muscle,
and superficial reflexes, which are elicited by stimulation of a sensory area,
are tested. The speed and strength of the reflex is assessed and usually
graded on a relatively crude five or six point scale. Differences in reflexes on
the two sides of the body are given special attention, as is the presence of
any pathological reflex such as Babinski's sign. The neurologist always makes
at least a superficial assessment of the patient's coordination and may test
coordination more specifically by having the patient carry out certain complex
actions. The presence of any abnormal movements such as tics, tremors, or
choreiform movements is always noted.

As with the motor examination, the extent of the sensory examination
may vary considerably, depending on the patient's complaint and other clinical
findings. A complete sensory examination involves assessment of sensations
of pain, temperature, touch, position, and vibration. Once again, the neurologist is particularly concerned with differences in these sensations on different
sides and different parts of the body.

Overall, the neurological examination is a process which often proceeds
in a successive screening manner. A history is always obtained and this dic-
tates to some extent the nature and extent of the physical examination. The
results of the various parts of the physical examination determine the extent
to which other portions of the examination are carried out, and the overall
results of the physical examination determine to some extent the use of other
more specialized tests (described in Chapter 10).

It should be clear from this brief description of the typical neurological
examination that there are certain limitations and values inherent in this procedure. A major limitation is posed by the skill of the neurological examiner.
Many portions of the examination require subjective judgments and grading.
These are most obvious in the motor examination and the assessment of
reflexes, where relatively crude rating scales are typically employed. The
cooperation of the patient also poses another major limitation. Certain portions of the examination, such as the sensory examination, obviously cannot
be carried out adequately on an unconscious patient. The patient must also
have sufficient comprehension to cooperate with certain portions of the examination. He or she must, for example, be able to report accurately the sensations experienced during the sensory examination. The ability to do this will
obviously be influenced by factors such as intelligence, psychiatric condition,
and general willingness to participate and cooperate.

Compared to other diagnostic procedures, the clinical neurological examination has a major value in that it is noninvasive and therefore produces little or no risk to the patient, except for certain specialized procedures which are not generally utilized. For the most part, the examination involves little discomfort to the patient, and is relatively inexpensive when compared to other specialized procedures described in the next chapter.

Chapter 10

SPECIALIZED NEUROLOGICAL-RADIOLOGICAL TECHNIQUES

Just as the neuropsychologist should understand the nature of the clinical neurological examination, he or she should also understand some of the specialized neurological-radiological diagnostic techniques. The decision to utilize any of the specialized techniques is dictated by a number of factors. The most prominent among these are the indications from the neurological history and the clinical examination. The different procedures yield information about different parts of the nervous system and have different reliabilities and validities associated with them. There are also differences in availability for each procedure, often determined by the cost of the equipment and the specialized skills needed to utilize them.

The simplest, most readily available, and most widely utilized of these techniques is the ordinary x-ray. This procedure is inexpensive and has no morbidity/mortality rate or discomfort for the patient associated with it. It is most useful in identifying the nature and extent of damage to the skull due to head trauma, but has the lowest hit rate for identifying other types of neuropathological processes (Filskov & Goldstein, 1974). Electroencephalography (EEG) is also widely available, relatively inexpensive, and has no morbidity/ mortality rate or discomfort for the patient. The EEG is most often indicated when there is a history or suspicion of a seizure disorder, and is particularly useful in identifying the anatomical focus of the seizures. It is a relatively weak technique for identifying other types of neuropathological processes.

Electromyography (EMG) and nerve conduction studies, which are often done in conjunction with each other, are less readily available and more expensive. They do not, however, have any morbidity or mortality rates associated with them, although they do entail a mild to moderate degree of discomfort for the patient. EMG studies typically involve insertion of small needle electrodes into various muscles in order to assess electrical function of the muscles. Nerve conduction studies involve applying an electrical shock to various nerves and measuring the conduction rate when electrodes are applied at different points on the nerve. These studies are used to differentiate between neuropathic and myopathic disorders and to determine the extent of progression or rehabilitation in various conditions.

Examination of cerebrospinal fluid obtained through a lumbar puncture is widely available and inexpensive. There is some degree of discomfort to the patient with this procedure and some risk of headache following it, as well as a minor risk of infection, as would be expected with any invasive procedure. Increases in intracranial pressure, which may be noted by measurement of the pressure of the fluid at the time of withdrawal are pathognomonic. Even the gross appearance of the spinal fluid may indicate the presence of blood cells in the fluid (xanthrochromia), which is also pathognomonic. Ordinarily, the spinal fluid should be clear and colorless and any deviation from this appearance should lead to a strong suspicion of a lesion in the nervous system. Laboratory examinations of the spinal fluid are typically carried out to identify the presence of disease organisms which may indicate infection, such as meningitis or syphilis, and the study of the complex chemistry of the spinal fluid may contribute to diagnoses such as multiple sclerosis.

The procedures described above can all be carried out in an office or clinic setting. Angiography, however, is a more seriously invasive procedure and is carried out in a hospital setting. This involves the introduction of a radiopaque substance into an artery through a catheter. The femoral artery is often utilized. X-rays of the skull are then taken as the radiopaque substance circulates through the cerebro-vascular system. As would be expected when a foreign substance is introduced into the body, there is an associated morbidity/mortality rate (.065 according to Filskov & Goldstein, 1974). This procedure, however, is extremely valuable in visualizing any abnormalities or lesions of the vascular system. It may also demonstrate space occupying lesions which distort the structure of the vascular system.

Pneumoencephalography is also an invasive technique with a morbidity/mortality rate of .025 (Filskov & Goldstein, 1974). This procedure requires the removal of spinal fluid through a lumbar puncture and the injection of air with subsequent examination of the brain by x-ray procedures. This technique is most useful for visualizing distortions of the ventricular system resulting from space occupying lesions, atrophy, or hydrocephalus. A common complication of pneumoencephalography is a severe, prolonged headache.

The brain scan is a procedure in which a radioisotopic substance is introduced into an artery and the brain is subsequently scanned by a type of scintillation counter. There is a morbidity/mortality rate associated with this procedure since it involves introducing a foreign substance into the body. It is most useful in identifying neoplasms, the tissue of which absorbs more of the radioactive substance.

Other new neurological diagnostic vistas have been opened up by the expansion of computer technology. The best known of these is computerized axial tomography (CAT). In the CAT scan procedure, the brain or other part of the body is scanned by an x-ray as the beam source and film plate move in opposite directions. This is often done both with and without the injection of the contrast medium into the vascular system of the brain. The computer then reconstructs pictures of different "slices" through the brain (or other part of the body). These may be viewed by the radiologist on a TV screen and permanent photographs of them are made for further study. The technical details and history of this procedure have been described by Gordon, Hermann, and Johnson (1975). The pictures of the brain that are produced usually correspond to anatomical sections of significant structures such as different levels of the ventricular system. This technique is the most promising one currently available for detection of many types of lesions as small as one centimeter in size. As do all other radiographic techniques, the CAT scan relies on the difference in density between normal brain tissue and abnormal brain tissue to detect lesions. Since some lesions are identical in density to normal brain tissue, they may be missed by this technique. Limitations result from the necessary scanning time, which was quite lengthy with earlier machines, but is being reduced with successive generations of machines, and the degree of resolution in the resulting picture. Artifacts may result from patient movement and it is sometimes necessary to sedate patients in order to eliminate movement. Additionally, one can expect some risk of anaphylactic shock when a contrast medium is introduced into the vascular system.

Just as many new drugs are often heralded as miracle cures, new diagnostic procedures such as the CAT scan are often regarded as final answers. Messina (1977), however, has shown that the CAT scan is not the final answer to all diagnostic problems. He compared the CAT scans of 123 patients who had been studied within two months prior to death with the corresponding sections of their brains on autopsy following death. He reported that between 11% and 27% of patients were misdiagnosed. Furthermore, chemical and metabolic disorders cannot be detected on CAT scans.

Another problem with the use of CAT scans is the relatively low availability and high cost. This procedure, because of the expensive and complex equipment needed, is presently available only in major medical centers and the cost for each examination is currently in the range of $300. Availability and cost are, however, rapidly improving.

Other uses of x-ray and computer technology which are still experimental include the Positron Emission Tomography (PET Scan) and Nuclear Magnetic Resonance (NMR); however, radiologists have not been the only medical specialists to use computer techniques to enhance the value of their standard diagnostic procedures. Neurologists and ophthalmologists have also applied

computer technology to improve the power of electroencephalographic examinations. Sokol (1976) has reviewed the diagnostic use of visual evoked potentials. In this procedure, EEG recordings are made from the occipital area while
the patient is presented with visual stimuli. These may be flashes of light or
patterned visual stimuli. A lengthy series of stimuli (for example, 64 flashes of
light at a rate of one per second) is presented to the patient while EEG recordings are made. A computer averages the responses over the series of flashes
or patterned stimuli, and the resulting average response pattern is presented
via an oscilloscope. Various characteristics of the response pattern are mea-
sured and recorded by the computer, and a permanent tracing is made for
further measurement and study.

At present, this technique appears to have mainly experimental use, but
it shows promise in assessing visual acuity in patients who are unable to
cooperate with the usual procedures. One of the more promising uses of this
technique appears to be in the study of patients with small lesions of the optic
tracts, such as the plaques found in multiple sclerosis. Rushton (1975), for
example, reported that twelve of fourteen patients with multiple sclerosis showed
an abnormal latency on visual evoked potential.

Similar techniques have been utilized to study auditory responses. The
study of "auditory brain stem responses" has been reviewed by Starr and
Achor (1975). Both visual and auditory evoked potential studies are noninvasive, create no discomfort for the patient, and can be performed relatively
quickly. However, these procedures are not widely available and are still largely
experimental in nature.

From the preceding discussion it should be clear that each of these techniques has its own particular advantages and disadvantages. Ordinary x-rays,
angiograms, pneumoencephalograms, brain scans, and CAT scans all give
the physician a "picture" of the brain which may be invaluable in cases where
surgical intervention is indicated. Examination of the cerebrospinal fluid indicates changes in the chemistry of the fluid and the presence or absence of
disease organisms. EEG techniques, including evoked potential studies, dis-
close the pattern of electrical activity of the brain and may lead to identification
of locations of lesions. Conduction studies demonstrate the electrical activity
of peripheral nerves which may have various diagnostic implications. One
should note, however, that of the procedures described only electromyography gives direct evidence of the functional ability of the patient.

The neuropsychological examination, on the other hand, is a noninvasive
procedure which may suggest the presence of lesions of various sorts before
they can be detected by other techniques. The neuropsychological examination also has the major advantage of showing the effect which a lesion has
on the patient's ability to function in daily life. Most importantly, the neuropsychological evaluation identifies areas of intact functioning as well as those of
impaired functioning; this information is essential in planning treatment and
rehabilitation.

Neurological and neuropsychological techniques should be complementary rather than competitive. Neurological and radiological techniques are essential in pinpointing the location of most lesions and in facilitating surgical and other medical intervention. Neuropsychological techniques are vital in identifying the functional effects of lesions and in describing the areas of relatively intact functioning which are important in planning rehabilitation and treatment.

Chapter 11

CASE ILLUSTRATIONS

The following cases illustrate the methods described in an earlier section of this Guide for interpretation of data from the Halstead-Reitan Battery. Each of the questions listed in Chapter 3 is addressed from the perspectives of the four methods of inference (level of performance, pattern of performance, right-left differences, pathognomonic signs). Following each of the inferences drawn from the data are references to the hypotheses in each of the appropriate chapters on which these inferences are based. The data for each case is preceded by a description of the information that was available to the interpreter at the time of testing. In some cases, the interpretation was done "blind" to the neurological diagnosis. In these cases the eventual neurological diagnosis follows the blind interpretation. In other cases the neurological diagnosis was known prior to the time of testing. In these cases, the interpretation provided is based only on the Halstead-Reitan Battery data, even though other neurological data was available. Finally, there are some cases for which a definitive neurological diagnosis, made independent of the Halstead-Reitan Battery data, was never available. Such cases are fairly common in clinical practice and are provided to illustrate some of the more perplexing diagnostic dilemmas which may frequently be seen.

CASE NO. 1

This is a 19-year-old, white, single, left-handed male with twelve years education in special education classes who suffered a severe head injury in an automobile accident approximately three years prior to assessment. He was unconscious for several weeks following the injury and remained hospitalized for several months. Extensive retraining of motor skills was done at a rehabilitation center. At the time of testing, he was showing impulsive sexually aggressive behavior which had resulted in his psychiatric hospitalization. Surgical reports available at the time of testing indicated that he had suffered extensive damage to the left frontal and anterior temporal lobes as well as sustaining blindness in his left eye as a result of the injury. Since this history was available to the examiner, the question of whether there was brain damage or not was obviously a moot one. Instead, the question was whether the structural damage sustained was consistent with the behavior shown at the time of examination and what the implications of this damage were.

1) Is there cerebral impairment?

Level of Performance Indicators – From this point of view, it is noted that the following scores, which are the strongest indicators of the presence of brain damage, are all in the impaired range. These are the Halstead Impairment Index (.9), Category Test (75 errors), TPT Localization (4), and Trails B (340 seconds) (4-1). It is also noted that the Digit Symbol subtest score on the WAIS is the lowest of all of the WAIS subtest scores. This is the WAIS subtest which is most sensitive to brain damage (4-22).

Pattern of Performance – This method of inference does not shed a great deal of light on the first question in this case. One should note, for example, that the Verbal IQ and Performance IQ are virtually the same (4-14).

Right-Left Differences – First note that the time with the nondominant hand on the TPT is substantially slower than the time with the dominant hand. This results in a score of 1 for the dominant hand and a score of 3 for the nondominant hand on the profile sheet (see Chapter 4 for the expected relationship between the performance of the dominant and nondominant hands on the TPT). Next, note that the score on the dominant hand on the Finger Oscillation test is 37.8, while the score for the nondominant hand is 20. This difference clearly exceeds the expected 10% difference (Chapter 4) and results in a rating of 3 for the dominant hand and 4 for the nondominant hand on the profile sheet. Similarly, the Strength of Grip with the dominant hand is 61.3 kg., while the Strength of Grip with the nondominant hand is 41.6 kg. Once again, this difference clearly exceeds the expected difference. Finally, note that there were 10 errors with the right hand and 4 errors with the left hand on fingertip number writing on the Sensory Perceptual Examination. Even though this patient made numerous responses on this test with numbers which were not included in the instructions, and while this is probably due to inattention or lack of understanding of the instructions, the number of errors is clearly much greater on one side of the body than the other. From the perspective of right-left differences, then, it should be noted that there are four tests on which the right-left differences exceed the expectation for normal subjects.

Pathognomonic Signs – It is first noted that there are no pathognomonic signs shown on the Sensory Perceptual Examination. Turning to the Aphasia Screening Test, the data are not quite so clear. First of all, note that the patient is grossly deficient in reading, spelling, and arithmetic skills. In view of his limited education it is probably best to consider these as deficits which preceded

DATA SHEET

RESULTS OF NEUROPSYCHOLOGICAL EXAMINATION

Case Number: #1   Age: 19   Sex: M   Education: 12-Sp.Ed. Handedness: L

Name: _____   Employment: Unemployed   IMPAIRMENT INDEX: 0.9 *

WAIS (or WAIS-R)

VIQ	7 3
PIQ	7 7
FS IQ	7 3

Scaled Scores

Information	5
Comprehension	7
Digit Span	4
Arithmetic	3
Similarities	1 0
Vocabulary	1
Picture Arrangement	6
Picture Completion	1 0
Block Design	6
Object Assembly	9
Digit Symbol	1

MINNESOTA MULTIPHASIC PERSONALITY INVENTORY

(T-Scores)

? L F K Hs D Hy Pd Mf Pa Pt Sc Ma Si

CATEGORY TEST   7 5 *

TACTUAL PERFORMANCE TEST

Time — # of Blks. In
Dominant hand: 5.5 — 1 0
Nondomin. hand: 7.8 — 1 0
Both hands: 4.1 — 1 0
Total Time: 1 7.4 *
Memory: 7 *
Localization: 4 *

TRAIL MAKING TEST

Part A: 2 0 7 seconds   0 errors
Part B: 3 4 0 seconds   0 errors

SEASHORE RHYTHM TEST (correct)

Raw Score: 2 1   Rank: 1 0 *

SPEECH-SOUNDS PERCEPTION TEST

Errors: 2 6 *

FINGER OSCILLATION TEST

Dominant hand: 3 7.8 *
Nondominant hand: 2 0.0

STRENGTH OF GRIP

Dominant hand: 6 1 kilograms
Nondominant hand: 4 2 kilograms

REITAN-KLØVE TACTILE FORM RECOGNITION TEST

	Errors	Seconds
Dominant hand:	0	2 1
Nondominant hand:	0	3 4

SENSORY SUPPRESSIONS

Dominant:
Nondominant:

APHASIA SIGNS: Poor reading, spelling and mathematical skills. Right-left confusion.
Blind in left eye.
Bilateral finger tip agnosia (left greater)
Bilateral asteriognosis

NEUROPSYCHOLOGICAL ASSESSMENT PROFILE

Patient Name: ___Case #1___   Age: _19_ Sex: _M_ Education: _12 SpEd_ Handedness: _L_

Rating Equivalents of Raw Scores

Test	0	1	2	3	4	5
Impairment Index	0 — .2 .3 —	.4 .5 —	.6 .7 —	.8 — (.9) — 1.0		
Category Errors	≤ 25	26–52	(53–75)	76–105	106–131	132+
(TPT) Time–Dom.	≤ 4.7	4.(8–8).2	8.3–10	10 & 9–5 in.	10 & 4–2 in.	10 & 1–0 in
(TPT) Nondom.	≤ 2.6	2.7–4.5	4.6–6.1	6.(2–8.)8	8.9–10&10–6 in	10 & 5–0 in
(TPT) Both	≤ 1.5	1.6–2.7	2.8–3.7	3.(8–5.)2	5.3–10	10 & 0–9 in
(TPT) Total	≤ 9.0	9.1–15.6	15.(7–2)1	21.1–29.9	30 & 14–30 in.	30 & 0–13 i.
(TPT) Memory	10–9	(8–6)	5–4	3–2	1	0
(TPT) Localization	10–7	6–5	(4–3)	2–1	0 & mem > 0	0 & mem = 0
Rhythm Errors	0–2	3–5	(6–9)	10–13	14–18	19+
Speech Errors	0–3	4–7	8–14	15–25	26(–30)	31+
Tapping (No.)						
Dom. M	≥ 55	54–50	49–43	(42–3)7	31–20	19–0
F	≥ 51	50–46	45–39	38–28	27–16	15–0
Nondom. M	≥ 49	48–44	43–37	36–26	25–14	13–0
F	≥ 45	44–40	39–33	32–22	2(1–10)	9–0
Trails A (time)	≤ 19	20–33	34–48	49–62	63–86	(87+)
Trails B (time)	≤ 57	58–87	88–123	124–186	187–275	(276+)
Memory						
ST	27+	24–26	18–23	14–17	9–13	0–8
verbal) ½ Hr.	24+	20–23	15–19	9–14	4–8	0–3
% Ret.	99–100	85–98	69–84	51–68	32–50	0–31
ST	12+	10–11	8–9	5–7	2–4	0–1
figures) ½ Hr.	11+	9–11	7–8	4–6	1–3	0
% Ret.	99–100	84–98	66–83	45–65	25–44	0–24

Verbal IQ ___73___   WMQ _____   Performance IQ ___77___

APHASIA SCREENING TEST

Form for Adults and Older Children

Name:_____Case #1_____Age:__18__Date:_____Examiner:_____

1. Copy SQUARE	18. Repeat TRIANGLE
2. Name SQUARE	19. Repeat MASSACHUSETTS MASSATUSETTS
3. Spell SQUARE CAN'T SPELL	20. Repeat METHODIST EPISCOPAL
4. Copy CROSS	21. Write SQUARE
5. Name CROSS AN "X", A SQUARE, A CROSS	22a. Read SEVEN SELUERY
6. Spell CROSS CAN'T SPELL	22. Repeat SEVEN
7. Copy TRIANGLE	23. Repeat/Explain HE SHOUTED THE WARNING.
8. Name TRIANGLE	24. Write HE SHOUTED THE WARNING. CAN'T SPELL
9. Spell TRIANGLE CAN'T SPELL	25. Compute 85 – 27 =
10. Name BABY	26. Compute 17 X 3 = 15 X 3
11. Write CLOCK	27. Name KEY
12. Name FORK	28. Demonstrate use of KEY
13. Read 7 SIX 2 SLICK	29. Draw KEY
14. Read M G W GUM	30. Read PLACE LEFT HAND TO RIGHT EAR. PALICE LEFT TO RILT HAIR
15. Reading I	31. Place LEFT HAND TO RIGHT EAR
16. Reading II	32. Place LEFT HAND TO LEFT ELBOW

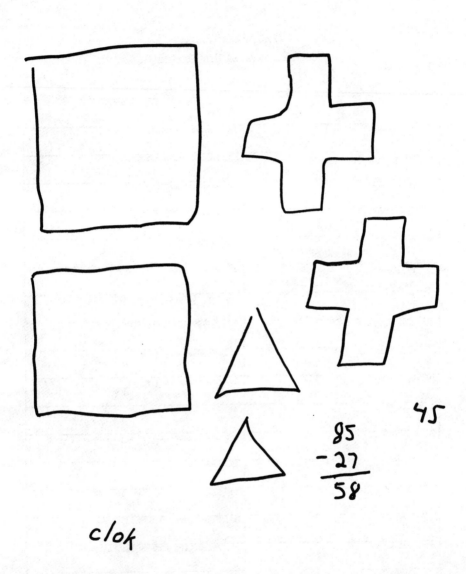

$$\begin{array}{r} 85 \\ -27 \\ \hline 58 \end{array}$$

45

clok

Case #1   SENSORY - PERCEPTUAL EXAMINATION

Indicate Instance in which stimulus is not perceived or is incorrectly perceived.

Tactile: Error
                                                                                  Totals

Right Hand-Left Hand - RH[   ]   LH[   ]   Both: RH[   ]   LH[   ]   RH_0_LH0_

Right Hand-Left Face - RH[   ]   LF[   ]   Both: RH[   ]   LF[   ]   RH_0_LF0_

Left Hand-Right Face - LH[   ]   RF[   ]   Both: LH[   ]   RF[   ]   RF_0_LH0_

Auditory:

Right Ear-Left Ear   - RE[   ]   LE[   ]   Both: RE[   ]   LE[   ]   RE_0_LE_0_

Visual:

Above eye level ⎰
Eye level   ⎱ RV[grid]   LV[grid]   Both:RV[grid]   LV[grid]
Below eye level

Finger Agnosia:

Right: 1[grid]   2[grid]   3[grid]   4[grid]   5[grid]   R 0/20
Left: 1[grid]   2[grid]   3[grid]   4[grid]   5[grid]   L 0/20

Finger-tip Number Writing Perception:

Right: | 4 6 3 5 | | 3 5 4 6 | | 6 5 4 3 | | 5 4 6 3 | | 6 3 5 4 | R 10 /20
Left: | 9 5 | | 8 | | 3   6 | | 3   7 5 | | 9 6 | L 4 /20
         | | | 5   1 | | 5   7 | | | | |

Astereognosis:

                | P N D | | D N P | Right: | N P D | R 2
Right: | P | Left: | P   D | Both: Left: | P | L 2

Tactile Form Recognition:

              | ○ □ △ ✛ | | △ ✛ ○ □ | | ✛ ○ □ △ | | □ △ ✛ ○ |
Errors: RH | |LH | |RH | |LH | |
                                                                         R 0
Response Time: | 5 4 5 4 | | 3 2 3 3 | | 4 3 4 5 | | 2 4 2 2 | L 0

                                    Total Time: R 34   L 21

Visual Fields: Left   Right

the head injury. (The patient reported 12 years of education, but it was noted that this was received in special education classes and probably reflects a long-standing learning disability.) There are, however, several items on this test which are noteworthy. First, on item 5, when asked to name a cross, the patient responded *"An X, a square,"* and only finally after a pause, *"a cross."* This type of hesitant, searching performance is characteristic of dysphasic responses. Similarly, items 13 and 14, on which the patient responded *"slick"* when asked to read "7-SIX-2" and *"gum"* when asked to read "MGW," probably cannot be explained by the educational history. Consequently, while it cannot be stated unequivocally that there are pathognomonic signs seen on the Aphasia Screening Test, there are at least these three items which are suggestive of brain damage (4-51).

In summary, it can be stated that the level of performance indicators and the right-left differences unequivocally point to the presence of brain damage. This conclusion would have been reached even in the absence of knowledge of the history available at the time of testing. With regard to the question raised in view of the history of an earlier injury, it can be said that these data clearly indicate that this man's injury resulted in significant behavioral deficits revealed by this testing. The pattern of performance method of inference was not helpful in this case, and the pathognomonic sign method of inference was somewhat equivocal.

2) What is the severity of brain damage?

Level of Performance – First, note the Halstead Impairment Index is .9, which is in the severely impaired range. An examination of the profile sheet, however, shows that the severity of impairment on individual tests ranges from none (TPT time-Dominant hand and TPT Memory) to severe (both Trails A and Trails B).

Pattern of Performance – As is usually the case, this method of inference yields little information regarding the question of severity.

Right-Left Differences – This method of inference also generally does not contribute a great deal to answering the questions about severity unless the differences noted are extreme. In this case, the differences appear to be moderate in degree on all of the tests where they are seen.

Pathognomonic Signs – The absence of pathognomonic signs on the Sensory Perceptual Examination indicates an absence of deficits which would be either medically significant or interfere with the patient's daily functioning. On the Aphasia Screening Test, the difficulties in reading, spelling, and arithmetic, while probably not pathognomonic signs, clearly present severe difficulties for this person's everyday functioning. The possible dysnomic and dyslexic errors noted on this test will also undoubtedly cause at least moderate difficulties in communication for the patient. Overall, the severity appears to be moderate with significant variations seen among functional areas.

3) Is the lesion progressive or static?

Level of Performance – First, note that the Full Scale IQ appears to be generally consistent with this man's educational background; however, the high Similarities and Picture Completion scores in comparison with other sub-test scores indicate a possible decline in cognitive abilities over time. Note that his performance on the Category Test, while in the impaired range, appears to be approximately consistent with his IQ (recognizing a moderate degree of acquired impairment). Finally, it can be seen that the performance on the Seashore Rhythm Test and Speech-sounds Perception Test does not rule out a progressive lesion (6-10).

Pattern of Performance – Note that the Verbal IQ and Performance IQ are virtually the same, which is unlikely in the event of a rapidly progressive lesion (6-8).

Right-Left Differences – As is usually the case, this method of inference yields little or no information regarding the question of velocity.

Pathognomonic Signs – No pathognomonic signs suggestive of a rapidly progressive lesion were noted. The possible dysnomic and dyslexic errors are clearly not severe enough to suggest any rapid progression.

In summary, this lesion is either static or, at most, only very slowly progressive.

4) Is the lesion diffuse or lateralized?

Level of Performance – This method of inference does not yield information regarding this question.

Pattern of Performance – Note that the Verbal IQ and Performance IQ are essentially the same, which would not suggest in and of itself any lateralization effect (5-2). It can be noted that the performance on the Speech-sounds Perception Test is considerably more impaired than the performance on the Seashore Rhythm Test. While this is, in itself, a weak indicator of lateralization, it is consistent with more impairment of the left cerebral hemisphere (5-13).

Right-Left Differences – As noted earlier, the performance on the TPT, Finger Oscillation Test, Strength of Grip and fingertip number writing all show differences which exceed expectations. Furthermore, it should be noted that all of these differences are in a direction which indicates a greater degree of impairment of the left cerebral hemisphere. Also note that there are 10 errors on the right hand on fingertip number writing test. This also is consistent with lateralization of damage to the left cerebral hemisphere (Chapter 4).

Pathognomonic Signs – The indications of dysnomia and dyslexia on the Aphasia Screening Test were noted earlier. Both of these signs would indicate lateralization of damage to the left cerebral hemisphere (5-28).

In summary, with regard to the question of lateralization, all of the data clearly implicate the left cerebral hemisphere as significantly more impaired than the right cerebral hemisphere, although there are some signs of right hemisphere impairment.

5) Is the impairment in the anterior or posterior part of the cerebral hemisphere?

Level of Performance – This method of inference does not yield information regarding this question.

Pattern of Performance – This patient's performance with his nondominant hand on the Finger Oscillation Test is more impaired than his performance with his nondominant hand on the TPT. This suggests a more anterior location of the lesion (5-34). It can also be noted that tactile performance on the Sensory Perceptual Examination is unimpaired with the exception of the errors on fingertip number writing. This also indicates a sparing of some of the more posterior portions of the left posterior parietal lobe (5-51).

Right-Left Differences – This method of inference does not yield information regarding this question.

Pathognomonic Signs – The Sensory Perceptual Examination, which showed an absence of pathognomonic signs, indicates a relative sparing of the more posterior portion of the cerebral hemisphere. On the Aphasia Screening Test, both expressive (dysnomia) and receptive (dyslexia) signs were seen. This would tend to implicate a fairly wide region in the anterior portion of the hemisphere.

The data, then, suggest that the lesion has affected principally the anterior portion of the left cerebral hemisphere and, furthermore, that the damage in this anterior region is fairly extensive, although it does not appear to extend into the posterior portion of the parietal lobe.

6) What is the most likely neuropathological process?

Reviewing the answers to the previous questions, the patient appears to have a moderately severe degree of cerebral impairment with the severity ranging from none in a few areas to severe in some other areas. The lesion appears to be static, or at least there is minimal evidence of any degree of progression. It is clearly lateralized to the left cerebral hemisphere with the anterior portions, including the frontal and temporal lobes, being most severely impaired. In spite of the clear-cut lateralization, there is evidence that the contralateral hemisphere is not spared from the effects of the lesion. For example, while the Finger Tapping speed with the dominant hand is severely impaired, the speed with the dominant hand is also impaired. This type of impairment of the contralateral hemisphere is seen in cases of intracerebral neoplasms, for example, in which pressure is exerted on the opposite side of the brain. In this case, however, the impairment of the contralateral hemisphere is more selective than one would expect in such cases, and a number of the tests are performed much too well to be consistent with that type of lesion (7-10). Another possible explanation for the impairment of the contralateral hemisphere would be the remote possibility of more than one lesion. This is statistically unlikely and, in general, one should attempt whenever possible to account for the data on the basis of a single lesion. Two such types of neuropathological processes in which multiple lesions occur simultaneously are multiple metastases and multiple sclerosis. The former of these can be ruled out on the basis that too many of the tests are performed well (7-15). Furthermore, metastatic carcinomas also show a pattern which reflects a much more rapidly progressive lesion than is seen in this case (Chapter 7). With regard to the possibility of multiple sclerosis, the impairment of the anterior portion of the left cerebral hemisphere appears to be too severe and widespread to be consistent with this. Multiple sclerosis typically does not become evident until a somewhat later age and severity of the degree shown here is rarely seen at this age. Furthermore, in multiple sclerosis one would expect to see more sensory impairment in at least one of the modalities (7-24). The other remaining possibility for explaining this limited damage to the contralateral hemisphere is that of the contrecoup effect seen in cases of closed head injuries (7-2). The most likely neuropathological process which would account for all of these data, then, is that of a severe closed head injury which may have occurred some time ago.

7) What are the implications for daily functioning and treatment?

It is clear that this person's sensory and motor abilities, while somewhat impaired, are adequate for daily functioning and probably also for some vocational adaptation. His problem-solving abilities, however, are quite impaired, and limit the range of vocational opportunities. Most importantly, his deficits in the basic skills of reading, spelling, and arithmetic indicate that he will need some degree of assistance in managing his daily affairs and will place significant limitations on his vocational skills. The impulsive, aggressive behavior noted in the referral question is quite likely related to the severe impairment of the frontal lobe.

The treatment recommendations included a major emphasis on a behavioral treatment program aimed at modifying his aggressive behavior. Intensive, individual instruction in basic academic skills was also provided. Assessment and preliminary training in a sheltered workshop revealed that this man was capable of performing simple, routine assembly tasks. The behavioral treatment reduced his aggressive behavior somewhat but did not eliminate it completely. Academic training met with limited success and he showed some slight improvement in this area. In a three year follow up, the patient continued to require a sheltered living situation due to his behavioral problems, although his adjustment was considerably improved and he was able to work daily in a sheltered workshop.

CASE NO. 2

This is a 58-year-old, white, married, right-handed male previously employed as an architectural engineer. Three years prior to testing, he had a small right parietal-occipital spontaneous intracerebral bleed which required a craniotomy for evacuation when it did not resolve spontaneously. According to the neurosurgeon, "post-operatively, he did well with improvement in his mental functioning and capability." A CAT scan a year later "showed evidence of previous craniotomy defect in the right parietal-occipital region but no other residual from that surgery was evident," and a neurologist's summary of his evaluation at about the same time indicated, "no significant neurological residual from the previous craniotomy." Two years following surgery, this man continued to be severely depressed, with prominent suicidal ideation, and was completely unable to work at his profession in spite of the fact that he had been given an essentially "clean bill of health" by both his neurosurgeon and neurologist. A neuropsychological evaluation was requested by the psychiatrist who was treating him for depression to "rule out organicity as the cause of this man's problems."

1) Is there cerebral impairment?
Level of Performance – Looking first at those best indicators of brain damage (4-1), the Halstead Impairment Index is .6, which is in the impaired range; the Category Test score is 85 and indicative of impairment; TPT Localization is 5.0, which is not impaired; and Trails B time is 105 seconds, which is in the impaired range. Thus, three of the four tests which are most sensitive to brain damage are in the impaired range. Also note that the Digit Symbol subtest scale score of 7 on the WAIS is the lowest of all of the WAIS subtest scores, and that this is the WAIS subtest which is most sensitive to brain damage (4-22).

Pattern of Performance – Note that this man has a Verbal IQ of 124 and Performance IQ of 110. This difference would generally not be considered a significant one, but in a man who has functioned for years as a successful architectural engineer, it is surprising that the Performance IQ is 14 points lower than the Verbal IQ. Consequently, the presence of brain damage is suspected.

Right-Left Differences – On the TPT, note that the time with the nondominant hand is slower than the time with the dominant hand, which is contrary to expectation (Chapter 4). Also note that the speed with the nondominant hand on the Finger Oscillation test is slower than expectation in relation to the speed with the dominant hand, resulting in a score of 2 for the dominant hand and a score of 3 for the nondominant hand. Similarly, note that the Strength of Grip with the nondominant hand (31.3 kg.) is greater than 10% weaker than that of the dominant hand (39 kg.) Both of these differences exceed expectations (Chapter 4). There were no significant differences in the functioning of the two sides of the body on the Sensory Perceptual Exam. Thus, from the perspective of this method of inference, three of the tests showed right-left differences which exceed the normal expectations; therefore, the presence of brain damage is strongly suggested.

Pathognomonic Signs – Both the Aphasia Screening Test and the Sensory Perceptual Examination are unremarkable with regard to pathognomonic signs.

DATA SHEET

RESULTS OF NEUROPSYCHOLOGICAL EXAMINATION

Case Number: __2__   Age: __58__   Sex: __M__   Education: __16+__   Handedness: __R__

Name: _____   Employment: __Engineer__   IMPAIRMENT INDEX: __0.6__ *

WAIS (or WAIS-R)

VIQ	1 2 4
PIQ	1 1 0
FS IQ	1 1 9

Scaled Scores

Information	1 4
Comprehension	1 4
Digit Span	1 4
Arithmetic	1 0
Similarities	1 4
Vocabulary	1 4
Picture Arrangement	8
Picture Completion	1 1
Block Design	9
Object Assembly	1 0
Digit Symbol	7

MINNESOTA MULTIPHASIC PERSONALITY
INVENTORY

(T-Scores)

?	
L	
F	
K	
Hs	
D	
Hy	
Pd	
Mf	
Pa	
Pt	
Sc	
Ma	
Si	

CATEGORY TEST   8 5 *

TACTUAL PERFORMANCE TEST

Time —— # of Blks. In

Dominant hand:	9 . 3	— 1 0
Nondomin. hand:	9 . 9	— 1 0
Both hands:	5 . 2	— 1 0

Total Time: 2 4 . 4 *
Memory: 7 *
Localization: 5 *

TRAIL MAKING TEST

Part A: 5 3 seconds   0 errors
Part B: 1 0 5 seconds   0 errors

SEASHORE RHYTHM TEST (correct)

Raw Score: 2 3   Rank: 9 *

SPEECH-SOUNDS PERCEPTION TEST

Errors: 7 *

FINGER OSCILLATION TEST

Dominant hand: 4 3 . 0 *
Nondominant hand: 3 6 . 2

STRENGTH OF GRIP

Dominant hand: 3 9 kilograms
Nondominant hand: 3 1 kilograms

REITAN-KLØVE TACTILE FORM RECOGNITION TEST

	Errors	Seconds
Dominant hand:	0	1 1
Nondominant hand:	0	1 2

SENSORY SUPPRESSIONS

Dominant: 0
Nondominant: 0

APHASIA SIGNS:
                    ·None

NEUROPSYCHOLOGICAL ASSESSMENT PROFILE

Patient Name: __Case #2__   Age: __58__ Sex: __M__ Education: __16+__ Handedness: __R__

Rating Equivalents of Raw Scores

Test	0	1	2	3	4	5
Impairment Index	0 — .2 .3 —	.4 .5 —	(.6) .7 —	.8 .9 —	1.0	
Category Errors	≤ 25	26-52	53-75	(76-105)	106-131	132+
(TPT) Time-Dom.	≤ 4.7	4.8-8.2	8(9-10)	10 & 9-5 in.	10 & 4-2 in.	10 & 1-0 in
(TPT) Nondom.	≤ 2.6	2.7-4.5	4.6-6.1	6.2-8.8	8.9-(10&10)-6 in	10 & 5-0 in
(TPT) Both	≤ 1.5	1.6-2.7	2.8-3.7	(3.8-5.2)	5.3-10	10 & 0-9 in
(TPT) Total	≤ 9.0	9.1-15.6	15.7-21	(22.1-29.9)	30 & 14-30 in.	30 & 0-13 i
(TPT) Memory	10-9	(8-6)	5-4	3-2	1	0
(TPT) Localization	10-7	(6-5)	4-3	2-1	0 & mem > 0	0 & mem = 0
Rhythm Errors	0-2	3-5	(6-9)	10-13	14-18	19+
Speech Errors	0-3	(4-7)	8-14	15-25	26-30	31+
Tapping (No.)						
Dom. M	≥ 55	54-50	(49-43)	42-32	31-20	19-0
F	≥ 51	50-46	45-39	38-28	27-16	15-0
Nondom. M	≥ 49	48-44	43-37	(36-26)	25-14	13-0
F	≥ 45	44-40	39-33	(32-22)	21-10	9-0
Trails A (time)	≤ 19	20-33	34-48	(49-62)	63-86	87+
Trails B (time)	≤ 57	58-87	(88-123)	124-186	187-275	276+
Memory						
ST	27+	24-26	18-23	14-17	9-13	0-8
verbal) ¼ Hr.	24+	20-23	15-19	9-14	4-8	0-3
% Ret.	99-100	85-98	69-84	51-68	32-50	0-31
ST	12+	10-11	8-9	5-7	2-4	0-1
figures) ½ Hr.	11+	9-11	7-8	4-6	1-3	0
% Ret.	99-100	84-98	66-83	45-65	25-44	0-24

Verbal IQ ___124___   WMQ _____   Performance IQ ___110___

APHASIA SCREENING TEST

Form for Adults and Older Children

Name:_____Case #2_____ Age: 58 Date:_____ Examiner:_____

1. Copy SQUARE	18. Repeat TRIANGLE
2. Name SQUARE	19. Repeat MASSACHUSETTS
3. Spell SQUARE	20. Repeat METHODIST EPISCOPAL
4. Copy CROSS	21. Write SQUARE
5. Name CROSS	22a. Read SEVEN
6. Spell CROSS	22. Repeat SEVEN
7. Copy TRIANGLE	23. Repeat/Explain HE SHOUTED THE WARNING.
8. Name TRIANGLE	24. Write HE SHOUTED THE WARNING.
9. Spell TRIANGLE	25. Compute 85 - 27 =
10. Name BABY	26. Compute 17 X 3 =
11. Write CLOCK	27. Name KEY
12. Name FORK	28. Demonstrate use of KEY
13. Read 7 SIX 2	29. Draw KEY
14. Read M G W	30. Read PLACE LEFT HAND TO RIGHT EAR.
15. Reading I	31. Place LEFT HAND TO RIGHT EAR
16. Reading II	32. Place LEFT HAND TO LEFT ELBOW

CASE #2

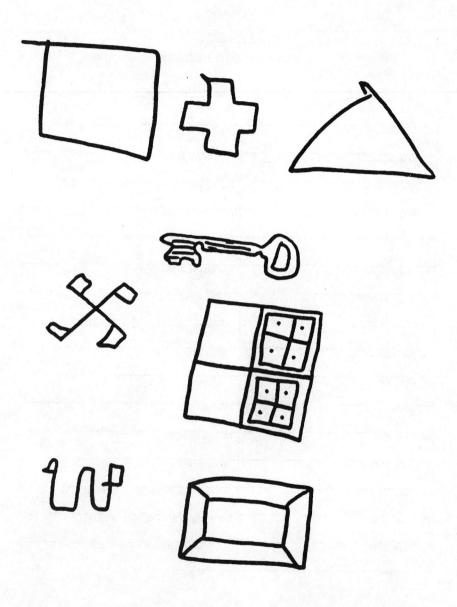

Case #2   SENSORY - PERCEPTUAL EXAMINATION

Indicate Instance in which stimulus is not perceived or is incorrectly perceived.

Error
Totals
Tactile:

Right Hand-Left Hand - RH[   ]   LH[   ]   Both: RH[   ]   LH[   ]   RH_0_ LH_0_

Right Hand-Left Face - RH[   ]   LF[   ]   Both: RH[   ]   LF[   ]   RH_0_ LF_0_

Left Hand-Right Face - LH[   ]   RF[   ]   Both: LH[   ]   RF[   ]   RF_0_ LH_0_

Auditory:

Right Ear-Left Ear   - RE[   ]   LE[   ]   Both: RE[   ]   LE[   ]   RE_0_ LE_0_

Visual:

Above eye level ⎧
Eye level   ⎨ RV[   ] LV[   ]   Both:RV[   ] LV[   ]
Below eye level ⎩

Finger Agnosia:

Right: 1[   ] 2[   ] 3[   ] 4[   ] 5[   ]   R _0_/ 20
Left: 1[   ] 2[   ] 3[   ] 4[   ] 5[   ]   L _0_/ 20

Finger-tip Number Writing Perception:

Right: [4|6|3|5] [3|5|4|6] [6|5|4|3] [5|4|6|3] [6|3|5|4]   R 2 /20
Left: [|6| |] [|5| |] [| |3|] [| | |] [| | |] L 1 /20

Astereognosis:

         [P|N|D]   [D|N|P]   Right: [N|P|D]   R _1_
Right: [|N|]   Left: [| |] Both: Left: [|N|]   L _1_

Tactile Form Recognition:

Errors: RH [O|□|△|✛] LH [△|✛|O|□] RH [✛|O|□|△] LH [□|△|✛|O]   R _0_
Response Time: [1|1|2|1]   [1|1|1|3]   [1|1|2|2]   [2|1|2|1]   L _0_

                              Total Time: R _11_   L _12_

Visual Fields: Left   Right

                    (circle)   (circle)

In fact, the verbal aspects of the Aphasia Screening Test were performed without error; on the Sensory Perceptual Examination, the patient made two errors on the right hand and one error on the left hand on fingertip number writing, and one error on each hand on tactile coin recognition, with all other responses on the examination being normal. When looking more closely at the drawings of the square, cross, and triangle on the Aphasia Screening Test, however, the minor errors which would not ordinarily be considered dyspraxic appear significant in light of this man's professional history. The difficulties in closure on all three of these drawings are clearly deviant for such a person. Next, looking at the drawings on the Wechsler Memory Scale (Form 1), note that the reproduction of Figure A is incorrect in that the "flags" should be facing each other. Note on Figure B that the left half of the figure is incomplete, and that on the right-hand portion of Figure C, the inner rectangle is not displaced to the right as it should be. In the context of this man's background, these are considered to be definite signs of constructional dyspraxia. Consequently, this method of inference also supports the presence of cerebral impairment.

2) What is the severity of brain damage?
Level of Performance – First, note that the Halstead Impairment Index of .6 is in the moderately impaired range. There is considerable scatter among the tests with regard to severity of impairment, which ranges from none (TPT Memory and Localization, Speech-sounds Perception) to severe (TPT time-Nondominant hand). While a Category error score of 85 would usually be considered to be in the moderately impaired range, for a man with this educational background 85 errors is considered to represent a severe deterioration from his probable premorbid level of functioning. The constructional dyspraxic errors, while considered mild for many patients, are considered to be severe for a man with this particular professional background. Therefore, the overall level of severity appears to be moderate, but in specific areas of functioning, it is quite severe.
Pattern of Performance – Ordinarily, a 14 point discrepancy between Verbal IQ and Performance IQ would not be considered a severe discrepancy. In the case of a man who had functioned as an architectural engineer, however, it would have been expected that his Performance IQ may well have exceeded his Verbal IQ premorbidly, and this particular pattern of performance is considered to represent at least a moderate degree of severity.
Right-Left Differences – The discrepancy between a performance of the dominant and nondominant hands on the TPT noted earlier is certainly a significant one and would lead to a consideration of at least a moderate degree of severity of impairment. The differences noted on the Finger Oscillation and Strength of Grip Test are not so severe and would not contribute significantly to a determination of the answer to this question.
Pathognomonic Signs – As noted earlier, the constructional dyspraxic signs shown by this man need to be considered in the context of his background and in this regard should be considered quite severe.

3) Is the lesion progressive or static?

Level of Performance – This man's Full Scale IQ, although possibly somewhat lower than his premorbid level of functioning, is not such that it aids in answering this question. His performance on the Category Test raises at least a question of a progressive lesion. However, his performance on the Seashore Rhythm Test is just into the impaired range and his performance on the Speech-sounds Perception Test is quite adequate. These latter two scores alone lead to a rejection of the hypothesis that there is a rapidly progressive lesion. It seems much more likely that this is a static lesion (6-10).

Pattern of Performance – The discrepancy noted between the Verbal IQ and the Performance IQ in the context of this case would at least raise the question of whether this might be a progressive lesion. There are no other data relevant to this question with regard to pattern of performance.

Right-Left Differences – As is usually the case, this method of inference yields little or no information regarding the question of velocity.

Pathognomonic Signs – No pathognomonic signs were noted that would have a bearing on the question of velocity.

In summary, the preponderance of evidence points to a static lesion.

4) Is the lesion diffuse or lateralized?

Level of Performance – This method of inference does not yield information regarding this question.

Pattern of Performance – The score on the Seashore Rhythm Test results in a score of 2 on the profile sheet, while performance on the Speech-sounds Perception Test leads to a score of 1 on the profile sheet. This, again, is a relatively weak indicator of lateralization, but is more suggestive of right cerebral hemisphere impairment (5-13). Also note that Part A of the Trail Making Test is performed slightly more poorly than Part B, another weak right hemisphere sign (5-9).

Right-Left Differences – As noted above, the performance on the TPT, Finger Oscillation Test, and Strength of Grip Test are all deviant from normal expectations and are in the direction which implicates the right cerebral hemisphere as being more impaired.

Pathognomonic Signs – The constructional dyspraxia discussed earlier is a weak sign of lateralization of a lesion in the right cerebral hemisphere (5-14).

In summary, it seems very clear that all indications point to substantially more impairment of the right cerebral hemisphere than of the left. The strongest signs seen in the right-left differences are supported consistently with the weaker signs seen in the pattern of performance on the WAIS, Seashore Rhythm – Speech-sounds Perception relationship, and Trails A – Trails B relationship.

5) Is the impairment in the anterior or posterior part of the cerebral hemisphere?

Level of Performance – This method of inference does not yield information regarding this question.

Pattern of Performance – Note that the performance with the nondominant hand on the TPT is more impaired than the performance with the nondominant hand on the Finger Oscillation Test. This relationship suggests a more posterior location of the lesion (5-34). Also note that there was no significant evidence of tactile perceptual impairment on the Sensory Perceptual Examination, suggesting a lesion located further posteriorly in the right cerebral hemisphere (i.e., at some distance posterior to the postcentral gyrus).

Right-Left Differences – This method of inference does not yield information regarding this question.

Pathognomonic Signs – As noted earlier, this man's drawings of the square, cross, and triangle on the Aphasia Screening Test, as well as his reproduction of drawings on the Wechsler Memory Scale are considered to show significant evidence of constructional dyspraxia. This would again suggest a posterior location for the lesion (5-48). Perhaps the most important observation regarding the specific localization of the lesion in this case is the omission of the left side of the stimulus figure in Figure B of the drawings on the Wechsler Memory Scale. This appears due to a neglect to the left side of the stimulus. It is not as complete a neglect as is sometimes seen, but is probably best understood in this way. Neglect of the left side of the stimulus is frequently seen with lesions in the right parietal-occipital area (5-49). This type of unilateral neglect is frequently seen even in the absence of visual field defects. It was noted in this man's medical history that he had shown a homonymous hemianopsia immediately following the occurrence of the lesion, but this defect was absent on subsequent examinations, including this neuropsychological examination. It is clear, therefore, that the lesion in this case is located in the posterior portion of the right cerebral hemisphere, most likely in the parietal-occipital region.

6) What is the most likely neuropathological process?

Reviewing the answers to the previous questions, note that the patient has a moderately severe degree of cerebral impairment with many areas of functioning being relatively spared while the impairment is more severe in some rather focal areas. The lesion appears to be static and is definitely lateralized to the right cerebral hemisphere with the posterior portion of this hemisphere being most affected. Specifically, the parietal-occipital area seems to be the site of the lesion. The more anterior portion of the parietal lobe (postcentral gyrus) appears to be spared and the temporal lobe shows little evidence of significant impairment. A fairly focal, but somewhat severe, CVA in the parietal-occipital region could account for these data, and the age of this man is consistent with such a lesion. Since nondominant Finger Oscillation speed and Strength of Grip show only mild impairment, this may indicate that there has been some recovery from this lesion. This is, of course, quite consistent with the neurological and neurosurgical history presented, and the implications of this and the referral question are addressed in the next section.

7) What are the implications for daily functioning and treatment?

The dilemma experienced in this case by the referring psychiatrist can be appreciated. Although this is a man who has a documented neurological lesion, his neurosurgeon and neurologist have given him a "clean bill of health." From the psychiatrist's point of view, this tended to be supported by the absence of signs of an "organic brain syndrome" on the mental status examination. The man's above average intelligence was obvious and he showed none of the traditional signs of OBS on the mental status examination. Still, he remained depressed and incapable of carrying out his ordinary daily activities. The data from this evaluation, particularly the Category and Trail Making Tests, indicate that he undoubtedly has difficulties in problem-solving in new, complex situations. The most significant deficits in this man's behavior, however, are those visual perceptive and visual constructive abilities which would be of crucial importance in his functioning as an architectural engineer. This man's severe depression is clearly related to his awareness of his loss of these important abilities, and his resulting inability to function at his previous profession. The effects of the neurological lesion, although clearly not medically or surgically treatable, must be taken into consideration as a major factor in the etiology of his depression. Psychological treatment must focus on his grief over the loss of these abilities and all of the other resulting losses in status and meaning in his life. In addition, it should capitalize on his relatively well-preserved strengths which are seen in his verbal intelligence.

CASE NO. 3

This is a 47-year-old, white, married, left-handed male physician. Until about three years prior to his evaluation, this man had functioned as a physician in independent private practice. He had no known previous psychiatric or neurological history of significance. Over the past three years, his level of functioning had gradually deteriorated. He began relying more on his office help and colleagues for assistance in carrying out his practice, and gradually his dependence on others increased until he was completely unable to work. Over the next year he became increasingly depressed, lost weight, ceased to pay attention to his personal appearance and hygiene, and became socially withdrawn and noncommunicative. He was hospitalized in a psychiatric hospital and the subsequent referral question from his psychiatrist was one of differentiating between "organicity" and depression.

1) Is there cerebral impairment?

Level of Performance Indicators – Note that the Halstead Impairment Index (.9), Category Test (86 errors), TPT localization (0), and Part B of the Trail Making Test (276 seconds) are all in the impaired range. These are the scores

DATA SHEET

RESULTS OF NEUROPSYCHOLOGICAL EXAMINATION

Case Number: 3   Age: 47   Sex: M   Education: 20   Handedness: L

Name: _____   Employment: Physician   IMPAIRMENT INDEX: 0.9 *

WAIS (or WAIS-R)		
VIQ		1 0 5
PIQ		8 6
FS IQ		9 6

Scaled Scores

Information	1 5
Comprehension	1 0
Digit Span	9
Arithmetic	5
Similarities	1 2
Vocabulary	1 2
Picture Arrangement	6
Picture Completion	8
Block Design	7
Object Assembly	4
Digit Symbol	5

MINNESOTA MULTIPHASIC PERSONALITY
INVENTORY
(T-Scores)

?	0
L	6 0
F	9 2
K	4 7
Hs	4 5
D	7 5
Hy	5 3
Pd	7 7
Mf	5 7
Pa	8 8
Pt	6 5
Sc	9 8
Ma	5 3
Si	6 8

CATEGORY TEST   8 6 *

TACTUAL PERFORMANCE TEST

	Time	# of Blks. In
Dominant hand:	1 0 . 0 —	6
Nondomin. hand:	1 0 . 0 —	4
Both hands:	1 0 . 0 —	9

Total Time: 3 0 . 0 *
Memory: 4 *
Localization: 0 *

TRAIL MAKING TEST

Part A: 1 0 6 seconds   0 errors
Part B: 2 7 6 seconds   4 errors

SEASHORE RHYTHM TEST (correct)

Raw Score: 1 6   Rank: 1 0 *

SPEECH-SOUNDS PERCEPTION TEST

Errors: 6 *

FINGER OSCILLATION TEST

Dominant hand: 4 6 . 8 *
Nondominant hand: 4 9 . 9

STRENGTH OF GRIP

Dominant hand: 2 1 kilograms
Nondominant hand: 2 5 kilograms

REITAN-KLØVE TACTILE FORM RECOGNITION TEST

	Errors	Seconds
Dominant hand:	0	1 9
Nondominant hand:	0	1 4

SENSORY SUPPRESSIONS

Dominant: 0
Nondominant: 0

APHASIA SIGNS: 7 Errors - dysnomia,
dyslexia, dyscalculia,
right-left confusion

NEUROPSYCHOLOGICAL ASSESSMENT PROFILE

Patient Name: Case #3   Age: 47   Sex: M   Education: 20   Handedness: L

Rating Equivalents of Raw Scores

Test	0	1	2	3	4	5
Impairment Index	0 —.2	.3 —.4	.5 —.6	.7 —.8	(.9) —1.0	
Category Errors	≤ 25	26-52	53-75	(76-10⑤)	106-131	132+
(TPT) Time-Dom.	≤ 4.7	4.8-8.2	8.3-10	10 &(9-5)in.	10 & 4-2 in.	10 & 1-0 in
(TPT) Nondominant	≤ 2.6	2.7-4.5	4.6-6.1	6.2-8.8	8.9-10&10-6 in	10(& 5-0) in
(TPT) Both	≤ 1.5	1.6-2.7	2.8-3.7	3.8-5.2	5.3-10	10 & 0-9 in
(TPT) Total	≤ 9.0	9.1-15.6	15.7-21	21.1-29.9	30 &(14-30) in.	30 & 0-13 i
(TPT) Memory	10-9	8-6	(5-4)	3-2	1	0
(TPT) Localization	10-7	6-5	4-3	2-1	0 & mem > 0	0 & mem = 0
Rhythm Errors	0-2	3-5	6-9	10-13	(14-18)	19+
Speech Errors	0-3	(4-7)	8-14	15-25	26-30	31+
Tapping (No.)						
Dom. M	≥ 55	54-50	(49-43)	42-32	31-20	19-0
F	≥ 51	50-46	45-39	38-28	27-16	15-0
Nondom. M	(≥49)	48-44	43-37	36-26	25-14	13-0
F	(≥ 45)	44-40	39-33	32-22	21-10	9-0
Trails A (time)	≤ 19	20-33	34-48	49-62	63-86	(87+)
Trails B (time)	≤ 57	58-87	88-123	124-186	187-275	(276+)
Memory						
ST	27+	24-26	18-23	14-17	9-13	0-8
verbal) ½ Hr.	24+	20-23	15-19	9-14	4-8	0-3
% Ret.	99-100	85-98	69-84	51-68	32-50	0-31
ST	12+	10-11	8-9	5-7	2-4	0-1
figures)½ Hr.	11+	9-11	7-8	4-6	1-3	0
% Ret.	99-100	84-98	66-83	45-65	25-44	0-24

Verbal IQ   105   WMQ   Performance IQ   86

APHASIA SCREENING TEST

Form for Adults and Older Children

Name: Case #3   Age: 47 Date: Examiner:

1. Copy SQUARE	18. Repeat TRIANGLE
2. Name SQUARE A BOX	19. Repeat MASSACHUSETTS
3. Spell SQUARE	20. Repeat METHODIST EPISCOPAL
4. Copy CROSS	21. Write SQUARE
5. Name CROSS A PLUS SIGN	22a. Read SEVEN
6. Spell CROSS	22. Repeat SEVEN
7. Copy TRIANGLE A RECTANGLE	23. Repeat/Explain HE SHOUTED THE WARNING.
8. Name TRIANGLE	24. Write HE SHOUTED THE WARNING.
9. Spell TRIANGLE	25. Compute 85 − 27 = 112
10. Name BABY	26. Compute 17 X 3 =
11. Write CLOCK	27. Name KEY
12. Name FORK	28. Demonstrate use of KEY
13. Read 7 SIX 2 7 - S - I - X - 2	29. Draw KEY
14. Read M G W M G M	30. Read PLACE LEFT HAND TO RIGHT EAR.
15. Reading I	31. Place LEFT HAND TO RIGHT EAR
16. Reading II	32. Place LEFT HAND TO LEFT ELBOW LH TO R ELBOW

CASE #3

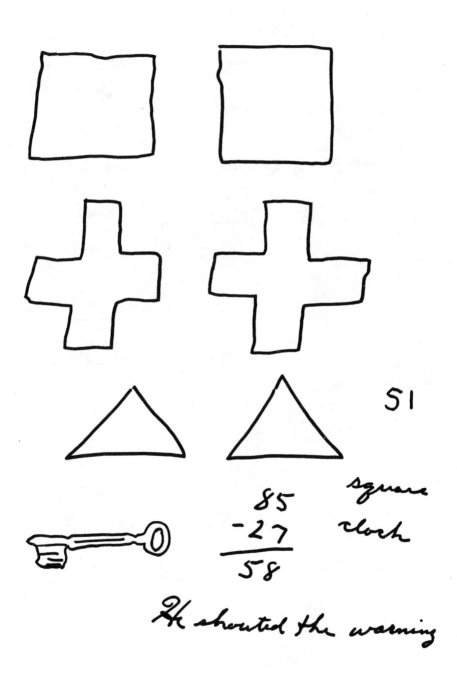

51

85
−27
―――
58

square
clock

He shouted the warning

Case #3

SENSORY - PERCEPTUAL EXAMINATION

Indicate Instance in which stimulus is not perceived or is incorrectly perceived.

Tactile: Error Totals

Right Hand-Left Hand - RH [ ] LH [ ] Both: RH [ ] LH [ ]   RH 0 LH 0

Right Hand-Left Face - RH [ ] LH [ ] Both: RH [ ] LF [ ]   RH 0 LF 0

Left Hand-Right Face - LH [ ] RF [ ] Both: LH [ ] RF [ ]   RF 0 LH 0

Auditory:

Right Ear-Left Ear - RE [ ] LE [ ] Both: RE [ ] LE [ ]   RE 0 LE 0

Visual:

Above eye level
Eye level   { RV [ ] LV [ ] Both:RV [ ] LV [ ]
Below eye level

Finger Agnosia:

Right: 1 [ ] 2 [X] 3 [ ] 4 [X] 5 [ ]   R 2 / 20
Left: 1 [ ] 2 [ ] 3 [X] 4 [ ] 5 [ ]   L 1 / 20

Finger-tip Number Writing Perception:

Right: [4 6 3 5 / 3] [3 5 4 6 / 6] [6 5 4 3] [5 4 6 3 / 3] [6 3 5 4 / 6]   R 4 / 20
Left: [2]   [6]   [6]   L 3 / 20

Astereognosis:

Right: [P N D / P] Left: [D N P / D] Both: Right: [N P D / D]   R 2
                                                Left: [N P D / D]   L 2

Tactile Form Recognition:

Errors: RH [O □ △ ✤] LH [△ ✤ O □] RH [✤ O □ △] LH [□ △ ✤ O]
Response Time: [2 1 2 2]   [3 2 3 2]   [2 1 2 2]   [2 2 3 2]   R 0
                                                                         L 0

Total Time: R 14   L 19

Visual Fields: Left   Right

which are most indicative of brain damage (4-1). The score on the Digit Symbol subtest of the WAIS (5) is the second lowest of all of the WAIS subtest scores. This is the subtest which is most sensitive to brain damage (4-22). This method of inference makes it clear that this man, with over 20 years of formal education, has suffered significant cerebral impairment.

Right-Left Differences – On the TPT, the patient placed six blocks correctly with the dominant hand, but only placed four correctly with the nondominant hand. On the Finger Oscillation Test, his finger tapping speed was actually slower with his dominant hand, and his Strength of Grip was weaker with his dominant hand. All of these relationships are deviant from normal expectations and are specific indicators of the presence of brain damage.

Pathognomonic Signs – The Sensory Perceptual Examination showed no pathognomonic signs, but this man made seven errors on the Aphasia Screening Test. The presence of any aphasia errors in the record of a man with this level of education is significant, and these should be considered to be pathognomonic signs of brain damage (4-51).

In summary, all four methods of inference clearly point to the presence of cerebral impairment in this case. This is a somewhat unusual case in that any one of these methods of inference, by itself, would have led to the same conclusion. As noted earlier, in many cases reliance on only one of the methods of inference often will not lead to a correct conclusion. In this case, the fact that all four methods of inference lead to the same conclusion serves to strengthen the conclusion that this man clearly has brain damage.

2) What is the severity of brain damage?

Level of Performance – First, note that the Halstead Impairment Index of .9 is in the severely impaired range. Furthermore, nearly all of the scores which contribute to this index are also in the severely impaired range. The Category score of 86 errors might be considered to be in the moderately impaired range for patients of average intelligence, but for a man with this educational background, this performance must be considered severely impaired. Of the scores which contribute to the Impairment Index only the TPT Memory, Speech-sounds Perception, and Finger Oscillation Test scores failed to fall in the severely impaired range. The scores on both Parts A and B of the Trail Making Test are also in the severely impaired range. It is clear that the degree of impairment in this case is severe.

Pattern of Performance – While this method of inference frequently yields little information regarding the question of severity, the 19 point discrepancy between Verbal and Performance IQs and the extreme scatter among the WAIS subtest scores indicates a severe degree of impairment.

Right-Left Differences – This method of inference also does not usually contribute to the answer of the question of severity, but in this case it is noted that on the TPT, Finger Oscillation Test, and Strength of Grip Test, the reversals from expectations are extreme. On the TPT, the patient actually placed fewer blocks with the nondominant hand, and on the other two tests his performance with the nondominant hand exceeded his performance with the dominant hand. Consequently, this method of inference also suggests a severe degree of impairment.

Pathognomonic Signs – As noted above, the presence of seven aphasia errors in a record of a man with this level of education is unusual and reflects a severe degree of impairment. It certainly would be consistent with his inability to function as a physician.

In summary, all four methods of influence make it clear that the overall level of impairment in this case is quite severe.

3) Is the lesion progressive or static?

Level of Performance – The Full Scale IQ, Verbal IQ and Performance IQ are all at a level which can be assumed to be considerably below this man's premorbid level. This raises doubts about a static condition and suggests that the possibility of a progressive lesion should be considered (6-7 & 6-8). His relatively good performance on the Speech-sounds Perception Test, however, makes a rapidly progressive, space-occupying lesion seem unlikely (6-10).

Pattern of Performance – This method of inference is not particularly helpful in answering this question in this case, although the substantial differences between Verbal and Performance IQs does suggest the possibility of a slowly progressive lesion.

Right-Left Differences – As is usually the case, this method of inference yields little information regarding the question of velocity.

Pathognomonic Signs – The absence of any suppressions on the Sensory Perceptual Examination makes doubtful the presence of a rapidly progressive space-occupying lesion.

The above inferences, along with the history of this man's deterioration over the past three years, leads to the conclusion that this is most likely a slowly progressive lesion (as opposed to a rapidly progressive, space-occupying lesion).

4) Is the lesion diffuse or lateralized?

Level of Performance – This method of inference does not yield information regarding this question.

Pattern of Performance – The difference between the Verbal IQ and the Performance IQ is suggestive of greater impairment of the right cerebral hemisphere. However, this finding should be tempered by both the fact that Performance IQ is generally more affected by damage to either cerebral hemisphere, and by the fact that this man's Verbal IQ appears to be substantially below its premorbid level (4-14). Note also that the performance on the Seashore Rhythm Test is substantially more impaired than performance on the Speech-sounds Perception Test. This is also a very weak indicator of lateralization of damage to the right cerebral hemisphere (4-43). Both of these weak indicators tend to point in the direction of more impairment of the right cerebral hemisphere, but are not conclusive in and of themselves.

Right-Left Differences – The performance with the nondominant hand on the TPT is less adequate than the performance with the dominant hand, which suggests left cerebral hemisphere involvement. Implicating the right cerebral hemisphere are the above noted differences on the Finger Oscillation Test and Strength of Grip Test. In addition to this, the time on the tactile form recognition test was somewhat slower with the dominant hand then with the nondominant hand, which also implicates the right cerebral hemisphere. These right-left differences clearly implicate both cerebral hemispheres with one strong sign (TPT) pointing to the left cerebral hemisphere and two others (Finger Oscillation and Strength of Grip) pointing to the right cerebral hemisphere. On the basis of right-left differences, it is difficult to say that this is a clearly lateralized lesion.

Pathognomonic Signs – The aphasia errors clearly indicate significant impairment to the left cerebral hemisphere (5-14).

In summary, strong indications of damage to both cerebral hemispheres are seen, with the TPT and aphasia signs particularly implicating the left cerebral hemisphere, and the Finger Oscillation and Strength of Grip performances most clearly involving the right cerebral hemisphere. On balance, it must be concluded that this is a pattern of diffuse or bilateral impairment.

5) Is the impairment in the anterior or posterior part of the cerebral hemisphere?

Level of Performance – This method of inference does not yield information regarding this question.

Pattern of Performance – The performance on the TPT is substantially more impaired than performance on the Finger Oscillation Test, which would suggest that involvement of the posterior portion of the hemispheres is greater than in the anterior portion (5-34). On the other hand, this man's very poor performance on the Trail Making Test and Category Test suggest the strong possibility of frontal lobe impairment (5-37). Overall, it seems that it is not possible to localize impairment within the cerebral hemispheres in this case.

Right-Left Differences – This method of inference does not yield information regarding this question.

Pathognomonic Signs – There were no pathognomonic signs seen on the Sensory Perceptual Examination and signs on the Aphasia Screening Test such as dyscalculia, dysnomia, dyslexia, and right-left confusion do not help substantially in answering this question.

Overall, it is not possible to localize the impairment either anteriorly or posteriorly within the cerebral hemispheres.

6) What is the most likely neuropathological process?

A review of the answers to the previous questions indicates a severe, probably slowly progressive, diffuse lesion in a 47-year-old man. This rules out several major categories of neuropathological processes which would show more lateralized pictures. There is a need to consider, then, the range of possibilities among the diffuse degenerative processes. The possibility of alcoholic deterioration seems unlikely on the basis of the history alone, which showed a deterioration over a period of two to three years. The severity of impairment along with this history is not consistent with alcoholic deterioration. Parkinson's disease can be excluded on the basis of the pattern shown on the profile, which is not consistent with this disorder; there is too much deterioration in IQ and not enough evidence of motor impairment (7-24). There remain two major possibilities, either hydrocephalus or cortical atrophy attributed to primary degenerative disease such as Alzheimer's type. It is not possible on the basis of this data to differentiate between these two processes, but a CAT scan and lumbar puncture should be helpful in making such a differential diagnosis. It should be noted that this can be a critical differentiation, because in some cases of hydrocephalus, neurosurgical procedures (shunting) are helpful.

7) What are the implications for daily functioning and treatment?

It is very clear that this man's ability to function in his previous profession is completely lost. On the other hand, his sensory and motor functions appear to be adequate for basic self-care skills such as bathing, dressing, and feeding himself. He appears to be able to communicate adequately with other people to meet his basic needs (the severity of his aphasic disorder does not seem likely to interfere with that). It is quite clear that this man will need a supervised living situation. Whether this needs to be in an institutional setting is dependent almost entirely on the degree of support that his family is capable of providing.

Two CAT scans completed on this patient revealed a "mild" degree of cortical atrophy and ruled out hydrocephalus. Turning to the original referral question of whether the diagnosis should be one of "organicity" or depression, the answer clearly is both. The primary diagnosis for this man is primary degenerative dementia with depression being secondary to his awareness of loss of functional abilities. On the basis of the CAT scan alone, without the neuropsychological evaluation, a diagnosis of primary degenerative dementia would probably not have been assigned. It is important to note that the CAT scan alone cannot be relied on to diagnose dementia.

In this case, with supportive psychotherapy and a behavioral treatment program, this man's self-care skills improved somewhat, although his mood remained significantly depressed. He was discharged from the hospital to a skilled nursing care facility.

CASE NO. 4

This is a 50-year-old white, divorced, right-handed female with 12 years of education who had operated her own bookkeeping business for a number of

DATA SHEET

RESULTS OF NEUROPSYCHOLOGICAL EXAMINATION

Case Number: 4   Age: 50   Sex: F   Education: 12   Handedness: R

Name: _____   Employment: Bookkeeper   IMPAIRMENT INDEX: 0.6 *

WAIS (or WAIS-R)

VIQ   8 8
PIQ   9 1
FS IQ   8 9

Scaled Scores

Information   7
Comprehension   6
Digit Span   9
Arithmetic   8
Similarities   8
Vocabulary   8
Picture Arrangement   7
Picture Completion   7
Block Design   9
Object Assembly   3
Digit Symbol   8

MINNESOTA MULTIPHASIC PERSONALITY
INVENTORY

(T-Scores)

?
L
F
K
Hs
D
Hy
Pd
Mf
Pa
Pt
Sc
Ma
Si

CATEGORY TEST   1 1 4 *

TACTUAL PERFORMANCE TEST

                        Time —— # of Blks. In
Dominant hand: 1 0 . 0 — 9
Nondomin. hand: 6 . 6 — 1 0
Both hands: 4 . 5 — 1 0
        Total Time: 2 1 . 1 *
        Memory: 6 *
        Localization: 6 *

TRAIL MAKING TEST

Part A: 3 0 seconds   0 errors
Part B: 9 8 seconds   4 errors

SEASHORE RHYTHM TEST (correct)

Raw Score: 1 8   Rank: 1 0 *

SPEECH-SOUNDS PERCEPTION TEST

Errors: 3 *

FINGER OSCILLATION TEST

Dominant hand: 3 0 . 4 *
Nondominant hand: 2 9 . 6

STRENGTH OF GRIP

Dominant hand: 2 0 kilograms
Nondominant hand: 1 7 kilograms

REITAN-KLØVE TACTILE FORM RECOGNITION TEST

                    Errors   Seconds
Dominant hand: 0   1 7
Nondominant hand: 0   1 6

SENSORY SUPPRESSIONS

Dominant: 0
Nondominant: 3

APHASIA SIGNS:
                    1 error
            Moderate constructional dyspraxia

NEUROPSYCHOLOGICAL ASSESSMENT PROFILE

Patient Name: ___Case #4___   Age: _50_ Sex: _F_ Education: _12_ Handedness: _R_

Rating Equivalents of Raw Scores

Test	0	1	2	3	4	5
Impairment Index	0 –|– .2	.3 –|– .4	.5 –|– (.6)	.7 –|– .8	.9 –|– 1.0	
Category Errors	≤ 25	26–52	53–75	76–105	(106–13)	132+
(TPT) Time–Dom.	≤ 4.7	4.8–8.2	8.3–10	10 & (9–) in.	10 & 4–2 in.	10 & 1–0 in
(TPT) Nondominant	≤ 2.6	2.7–4.5	4.6–6.1	(8.2–).8	8.9–10&10–6 in	10 & 5–0 in
(TPT) Both	≤ 1.5	1.6–2.7	2.8–3.7	(3.8–).2	5.3–10	10 & 0–9 in
(TPT) Total	≤ 9.0	9.1–15.6	15.7–21	2(.1–).9.9	30 & 14–30 in.	30 & 0–13 i
(TPT) Memory	10–9	(8–6)	5–4	3–2	1	0
(TPT) Localization	10–7	(6–5)	4–3	2–1	0 & mem > 0	0 & mem = 0
Rhythm Errors	0–2	3–5	6–9	(10–1)	14–18	19+
Speech Errors	(0–3)	4–7	8–14	15–25	26–30	31+
Tapping (No.)						
Dom. M	≥ 55	54–50	49–43	(2–3)	31–20	19–0
F	≥ 51	50–46	45–39	(8–2)	27–16	15–0
Nondom. M	≥ 49	48–44	43–37	3(–6)	25–14	13–0
F	≥ 45	44–40	39–33	(2–22)	21–10	9–0
Trails A (time)	≤ 19	(0–3)	34–48	49–62	63–86	87+
Trails B (time)	≤ 57	58–87	(8–12)	124–186	187–275	276+
Memory						
verbal) ST	27+	24–26	18–23	14–17	9–13	0–8
½ Hr.	24+	20–23	15–19	9–14	4–8	0–3
% Ret.	99–100	85–98	69–84	51–68	32–50	0–31
figures) ST	12+	10–11	8–9	5–7	2–4	0–1
½ Hr.	11+	9–11	7–8	4–6	1–3	0
% Ret.	99–100	84–98	66–83	45–65	25–44	0–24

Verbal IQ ____88____   WMQ _____   Performance IQ ____91____

APHASIA SCREENING TEST

Form for Adults and Older Children

Name:___Case #4_____   Age:__50__Date:_____Examiner:_____

1. Copy SQUARE	18. Repeat TRIANGLE
2. Name SQUARE	19. Repeat MASSACHUSETTS
3. Spell SQUARE	20. Repeat METHODIST EPISCOPAL
4. Copy CROSS	21. Write SQUARE
5. Name CROSS AN "X"	22a. Read SEVEN
6. Spell CROSS	22. Repeat SEVEN
7. Copy TRIANGLE	23. Repeat/Explain HE SHOUTED THE WARNING.
8. Name TRIANGLE	24. Write HE SHOUTED THE WARNING.
9. Spell TRIANGLE	25. Compute 85 - 27 =
10. Name BABY	26. Compute 17 X 3 =
11. Write CLOCK	27. Name KEY
12. Name FORK	28. Demonstrate use of KEY
13. Read 7 SIX 2	29. Draw KEY
14. Read M G W	30. Read PLACE LEFT HAND TO RIGHT EAR.
15. Reading I	31. Place LEFT HAND TO RIGHT EAR
16. Reading II	32. Place LEFT HAND TO LEFT ELBOW

CASE #4

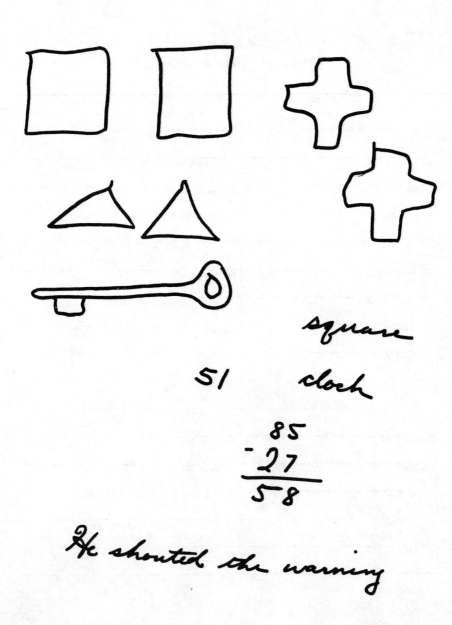

square

51   cloch

$$85$$
$$-27$$
$$\overline{58}$$

He shouted the warning

Case #4   SENSORY - PERCEPTUAL EXAMINATION

Indicate Instance in which stimulus is not perceived or is incorrectly perceived.

Error
Totals

Tactile:

Right Hand-Left Hand - RH[ ][ ][ ][ ]   LH[ ][ ][ ][ ]   Both: RH[ ][ ][ ][ ]   LH[ ][ ][ ][ ]   RH 0 LH 0

Right Hand-Left Face - RH[ ][ ][ ][ ]   LF[ ][ ][ ][ ]   Both: RH[ ][ ][ ][ ]   LF[ ][ ][ ][ ]   RH 0 LF 0

Left Hand-Right Face - LH[ ][ ][ ][ ]   RF[ ][ ][ ][ ]   Both: LH[X][X][X]   RF[ ][ ][ ][ ]   RF 0 LH 3

Auditory:

Right Ear-Left Ear - RE[ ][ ][ ][ ]   LE[ ][ ][ ][ ]   Both: RE[ ][ ][ ][ ]   LE[ ][ ][ ][ ]   RE 0 LE

Visual:

Above eye level
Eye level   { RV [grid]   LV [grid]   Both:RV [grid]   LV [grid]
Below eye level

Finger Agnosia:

Right: 1 [grid]   2 [grid]   3 [grid]   4 [X]   5 [grid]   R 1 / 20
Left: 1 [grid]   2 [grid]   3 [grid]   4 [grid]   5 [grid]   L 0 / 20

Finger-tip Number Writing Perception:

Right: 4 6 3 5 | 3 5 4 6 | 6 5 4 3 | 5 4 6 3 | 6 3 5 4   R 0 / 20
Left: L 0 / 20

Astereognosis:

Right: [P][N][D]   Left: [D][N][P]   Both: Right: [N][P][D]   R 0
                                           Left: [P]   L 1

Tactile Form Recognition:

Errors: RH [○□△✚]   LH [△✚○□]   RH [✚○□△]   LH [□△✚○]
Response Time: 3 2 2 2   4 4 3 2   2 2 2 2   4 3 2 2   R 0
                                                               L 0

Total Time: R 17   L 16

Visual Fields: Left   Right

[circle]   [circle]

years. At the time of her first admission to a psychiatric hospital, just prior to this evaluation, she was showing signs of agitated depression, alternating with grandiose ideas, and accompanied by poor judgment. She had recently lost several thousand dollars on a poorly conceived business venture. She had no previous history of psychiatric problems, and was referred by her psychiatrist for neuropsychological evaluation for assistance in arriving at a diagnosis.

1) Is there cerebral impairment?
Level of Performance – The Impairment Index (.6), Category score (114), and Trails B score (98) are all in the impaired range. These are three of the four strongest indicators of impairment (4-1). This woman's performance on the WAIS also indicates a decline from her previous level of functioning as indicated by her vocational history. This method of inference, therefore, supports the conclusion that there is brain damage.

Pattern of Performance – In this case, this method of inference is not helpful in answering this first question.

Right-Left Differences – The performance on the TPT is quite poor with both hands, but the relationship between the hands is about what would be expected. Similarly, the relationship between the two hands on Strength of Grip is about normal. Tapping speed with the dominant hand, however, does not show the expected 10% superiority over the nondominant hand. On the Sensory Perceptual Examination, the failure to perceive stimulation of the left hand when touched simultaneously with the right face, is also deviant (Chapter 4). These right-left differences clearly point to the presence of brain damage.

Pathognomonic Signs – The presence of even one aphasia error in the record of this patient is a significant sign. Even more notable is the record of the three suppressions seen on the Sensory Perceptual Examination. These data are strong evidence for brain damage (4-69).

2) What is the severity of brain damage?
Level of Performance – With the exceptions of the scores on TPT Localization and Memory, Speech-sounds Perception, and Trails A, all of the scores are in the moderately impaired range.

Pattern of Performance – This method of inference is not helpful in this case.

Right-Left Differences – The right-left difference on Tapping is only a slight one, but the difference seen on the suppressions on the Sensory Perceptual Examination is a significant one and indicates at least a moderate severity.

Pathognomonic Signs – The single aphasia error does not indicate a very high level of severity, but the suppressions point to a rather severe lesion (e.g., 7-11).

3) Is the lesion progressive or static?
Level of Performance – This woman's IQ appears to be somewhat lower than her premorbid level, but the decline is not great enough to support the inference of a rapidly progressive lesion. Her performance on the Seashore

Rhythm Test raises the possibility of a significant degree of progression, but her adequate score on the Speech-sounds Perception Test makes this less likely (4-40).

Pattern of Performance – This method of inference does not support a rapidly progressive lesion, since there is no difference between Verbal IQ and Performance IQ (4-16).

Right-Left Differences – This method of inference does not yield information regarding this question.

Pathognomonic Signs – The presence of three suppressions suggests the possibility of a tissue destroying lesion, which could be a progressive one (4-70). The absence of any history of past trauma to this woman's brain makes this seem quite likely.

Overall, the data yields a somewhat equivocal answer to this question. The possibility of some degree of progression cannot be ruled out. As is often the case, it would be very helpful to see the testing repeated at a later date in order to answer this question with a reasonable degree of confidence.

4) Is the lesion diffuse or lateralized?

Level of Performance – This method of inference does not yield information regarding this question.

Pattern of Performance – The lack of a difference between Verbal IQ and Performance IQ fails to support any lateralization (4-14).

Right-Left Differences – The difference between the two hands on Tapping indicates more impairment in the motor area in the left hemisphere, while the suppressions indicate more impairment in the sensory area of the right hemisphere. Considering both of these factors, it can be concluded that there is bilateral impairment.

Pathognomonic Signs – As indicated above, the suppressions indicate right hemisphere impairment; it can now be noted that the aphasia sign indicates left hemisphere impairment (4-51).

5) Is the impairment in the anterior or posterior part of the cerebral hemisphere?

Level of Performance – This method of inference does not yield information regarding this question.

Pattern of Performance – Since both cerebral hemispheres show impairment in this case, these must both be considered separately. In the left hemisphere, it is noted that the anterior (motor cortex) is impaired while the posterior (sensory cortex) probably is not, or at least is less impaired. In the right hemisphere, the posterior portion is significantly impaired as shown by the suppressions (4-70). It can be concluded, then, that the anterior portion of the left hemisphere is more impaired while the posterior portion of the right hemisphere is more impaired.

Right-Left Differences – This method of inference does not yield information regarding this question.

Pathognomonic Signs – In addition to the conclusions regarding the posterior portion of the right hemisphere, the aphasia sign suggests a more anterior (perhaps temporal lobe) impairment in the left hemisphere.

Once again, there is support for a pattern of right posterior and left anterior impairment.

6) What is the most likely neuropathological process?

To review the answers to the earlier questions, this is a case with moderately severe impairment and possible progressive velocity. There is bilateral impairment involving both hemispheres with more posterior impairment of the right hemisphere and more anterior impairment of the left one. The diffuse, degenerative processes can be ruled out because the focal areas of bilateral impairment appear too "sharp" or severe within the overall context. This picture leads to consideration of both multiple metastatic tumors and multiple sclerosis (Chapter 7). With multiple sclerosis, more sensory impairment (7-24) and less impairment of Verbal IQ would be expected (7-25). On the other hand, with a metastatic carcinoma, a much poorer performance overall would be expected (7-15). Considering all of these discrepancies, a strong possibility of a metastatic carcinoma was considered and a CAT scan recommended. At this point, the chest x-ray on this woman became available, and it revealed a large tumor. A biopsy of the tumor showed that it was highly malignant and of the type that frequently metastasizes to the brain.

7) What are the implications for daily functioning and treatment?

Unfortunately, the primary tumor was inoperable, and this patient was transferred to a nursing care facility where she died only a few months later.

CASE NO. 5

This is the case of a 65-year-old, white, right-handed male with 20 years of education, who was a retired pharmacist. Several years earlier, he had been diagnosed as having a right frontal glioblastoma (neoplasm) and subsequently had surgery three times for recurrence of this rapidly progressive neoplastic disease. He was referred by his neurosurgeon for a neuropsychological examination to determine the extent of recovery since his latest surgery (3 months previous) and his level of cognitive impairment, so that appropriate living conditions could be developed. Neurodiagnosis was not an issue, but rather how the brain damage was affecting his everyday functioning. To be certain that the Halstead-Reitan test results are delineating the cognitive and behavioral strengths and weaknesses associated with this disorder, an attempt to answer the questions associated with the brain damage issue will be presented first.

1) Is there cerebral impairment?
Level of Performance – All of the strongest indicators of brain damage are well into the impaired range; the Halstead Impairment Index is 1.0, the Category Test reflects 124 errors, TPT Localization is 0, and Trail Making B is

DATA SHEET

RESULTS OF NEUROPSYCHOLOGICAL EXAMINATION

Case Number: 5   Age: 65   Sex: M   Education: 20   Handedness: R

Name: _____   Employment: Retired Pharmacist IMPAIRMENT INDEX: 1.0 *

WAIS (or WAIS-R)

VIQ	1 1 6
PIQ	8 2
FS IQ	1 0 2

Scaled Scores

Information	1 2
Comprehension	1 6
Digit Span	9
Arithmetic	7
Similarities	1 2
Vocabulary	1 4
Picture Arrangement	4
Picture Completion	4
Block Design	5
Object Assembly	5
Digit Symbol	3

MINNESOTA MULTIPHASIC PERSONALITY
INVENTORY

(T-Scores)

?	
L	
F	
K	
Hs	
D	
Hy	
Pd	
Mf	
Pa	
Pt	
Sc	
Ma	
Si	

CATEGORY TEST   1 2 4 *

TACTUAL PERFORMANCE TEST

Time —— # of Blks. In

	Time		# of Blks. In
Dominant hand:	1 0 . 0	—	2
Nondomin. hand:	1 0 . 0	—	3
Both hands:	1 0 . 0	—	3

Total Time: 3 0 . 8 *
Memory: 7 *
Localization: 0 *

TRAIL MAKING TEST

Part A: 1 2 2 seconds   0 errors
Part B: 3 0 0 seconds   3 errors

SEASHORE RHYTHM TEST (correct)

Raw Score: 1 6   Rank: 1 0 *

SPEECH-SOUNDS PERCEPTION TEST

Errors: 2 9 *

FINGER OSCILLATION TEST

Dominant hand: 4 4 . 0 *
Nondominant hand: 2 7 . 0

STRENGTH OF GRIP

Dominant hand: 3 6 kilograms
Nondominant hand: 2 1 kilograms

REITAN-KLØVE TACTILE FORM RECOGNITION TEST

	Errors	Seconds
Dominant hand:	0	4 6
Nondominant hand:	0	9 9

SENSORY SUPPRESSIONS

Dominant: 8
Nondominant: 9

APHASIA SIGNS: Dysnomia, right-left
                       confusion.

NEUROPSYCHOLOGICAL ASSESSMENT PROFILE

Patient Name: ___Case #5___   Age: _65_ Sex: _M_ Education: _20_ Handedness: _R_

Rating Equivalents of Raw Scores

Test	0	1	2	3	4	5
Impairment Index	0 —|- .2 .3 -|- .4 .5 -|- .6 .7 -|- .8 .9 —|- (.0)					
Category Errors	≤ 25	26-52	53-75	76-105	(106-13)	132+
(TPT) Time-Dom.	≤ 4.7	4.8-8.2	8.3-10	10 & 9-5 in.	10 & 4-2 in.	10 & 1-0 in.
(TPT) Nondominant	≤ 2.6	2.7-4.5	4.6-6.1	6.2-8.8	8.9-10&10-6 in	(10 & 5-0 in.)
(TPT) Both	≤ 1.5	1.6-2.7	2.8-3.7	3.8-5.2	5.3-10	(10 & 0-9 in.)
(TPT) Total	≤ 9.0	9.1-15.6	15.7-21	21.1-29.9	30 & 14-30 in.	(30 & 0-13 i:)
(TPT) Memory	10-9	8-6	5-4	(3-2)	1	0
(TPT) Localization	10-7	6-5	4-3	2-1	(0 & mem) 0	0 & mem = 0
Rhythm Errors	0-2	3-5	6-9	10-13	14-18	(19+)
Speech Errors	0-3	4-7	8-14	15-25	26-30	(31+)
Tapping (No.)						
Dom. M	≥ 55	54-50	(49-4?)	42-32	31-20	19-0
F	≥ 51	50-46	45-39	38-28	27-16	15-0
Nondom. M	≥ 49	48-44	43-37	(36-2?)	25-14	13-0
F	≥ 45	44-40	39-33	(32-2?)	21-10	9-0
Trails A (time)	≤ 19	20-33	34-48	49-62	63-86	(87+)
Trails B (time)	≤ 57	58-87	88-123	124-186	187-275	(276+)
Memory						
ST	27+	24-26	18-23	14-17	9-13	0-8
verbal) ½ Hr.	24+	20-23	15-19	9-14	4-8	0-3
% Ret.	99-100	85-98	69-84	51-68	32-50	0-31
ST	12+	10-11	8-9	5-7	2-4	0-1
figures)½ Hr.	11+	9-11	7-8	4-6	1-3	0
% Ret.	99-100	84-98	66-83	45-65	25-44	0-24

Verbal IQ ___116___   WMQ_____   Performance IQ ___82___

APHASIA SCREENING TEST

Form for Adults and Older Children

Name: _____ Case #5 _____ Age: _65_ Date: _____ Examiner: _____

1. Copy SQUARE	18. Repeat TRIANGLE
2. Name SQUARE	19. Repeat MASSACHUSETTS MASSACHUSESS
3. Spell SQUARE	20. Repeat METHODIST EPISCOPAL
4. Copy CROSS	21. Write SQUARE
5. Name CROSS A STAR OR A RECTANGLE-NAZI INSIGNIA	22a. Read SEVEN
6. Spell CROSS	22. Repeat SEVEN
7. Copy TRIANGLE	23. Repeat/Explain HE SHOUTED THE WARNING.
8. Name TRIANGLE	24. Write HE SHOUTED THE WARNING.
9. Spell TRIANGLE	25. Compute 85 − 27 =
10. Name BABY	26. Compute 17 X 3 =
11. Write CLOCK	27. Name KEY
12. Name FORK	28. Demonstrate use of KEY
13. Read 7 SIX 2	29. Draw KEY
14. Read M G W M-G-M	30. Read PLACE LEFT HAND TO RIGHT EAR. RIGHT HAND TO RIGHT EAR - LOOKS CONFUSED
15. Reading I	31. Place LEFT HAND TO RIGHT EAR
16. Reading II	32. Place LEFT HAND TO LEFT ELBOW

CASE #5

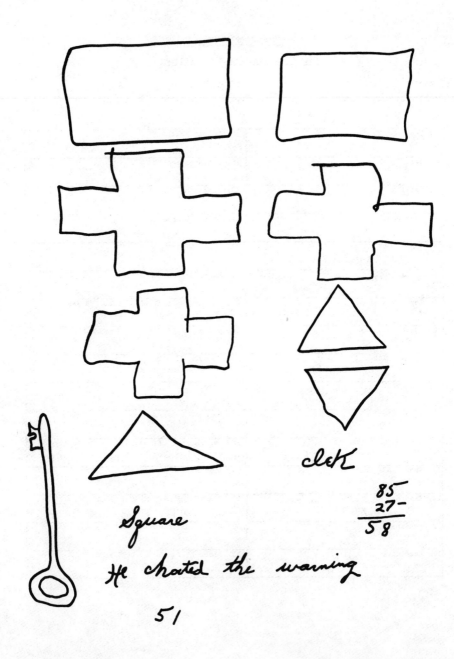

Case #5   SENSORY - PERCEPTUAL EXAMINATION

Indicate Instance in which stimulus is not perceived or is incorrectly perceived.

Tactile: Error
                                                                                  Totals

Right Hand-Left Hand - RH[   ]   LH[   ]   Both: RH[X| |X|] LH[X|X|] RH 2 LH 2

Right Hand-Left Face - RH[   ]   LF[   ]   Both: RH[|X|X|] LF[X| |X|X] RH 2 LF 3

Left Hand-Right Face - LH[   ]   RF[   ]   Both: LH[| |X|] RF[X|X|] RF 2 LH 1

Auditory:

Right Ear-Left Ear   - RE[   ]   LE[   ]   Both: RE[|X|X|] LE[X| |X|] RE 2 LE 2

Visual:

Above eye level   ⎧
Eye level   ⎨ RV [grid]   LV [grid]   Both:RV [grid, X above]   LV [grid]
Below eye level   ⎩

Finger Agnosia:

Right: 1[grid] 2[X] 3[X] 4[X] 5[grid]   R 3 /20
Left: 1[grid] 2[ ] 3[ ] 4[X|X] 5[grid]   L 4 /20

Finger-tip Number Writing Perception:

Right: [4|6|3|5 / 5] [3|5|4|6 / 3] [6|5|4|3 / 6] [5|4|6|3 / 5] [6|3|5|4 / 3]   R 3 /20
Left: [| | |6]   L 3 /20

Astereognosis:

Right: [P|N|D / N]   Left: [D|N|P / P]   Both: Right: [N|P|D /] R 1
                                                  Left: [P| |]   L 2

Tactile Form Recognition:

Errors: RH [O□△✚] LH [△✚O□] RH [✚O□△] LH [□△✚O]   R 0
Response Time: [4|6|7|4] [17|14|13|15] [5|4|7|9] [11|12|9|8]   L 0

                    Total Time: R 46   L 99

Visual Fields: Left   Right
                    [circle]   [circle]

greater than 300 seconds with three errors (4-1). Also note that Digit Symbol on the WAIS is the lowest subtest score, which is consistent with indications of cerebral impairment (4-22).

Pattern of Performance – The WAIS Verbal and Performance IQ discrepancy of 34 points suggests brain damage, specifically lateralization to the right cerebral hemisphere (4-14). The extremely low scores on the subtests of the Performance section are indicative of a decline from a previously higher level of mental functioning, since it is doubtful that an individual could complete the graduate education necessary to become a pharmacist with such poor visuospatial problem-solving skills.

Right-Left Differences – This patient was unable to complete the TPT, which supports the diagnosis of brain damage. He also demonstrated bilateral, yet primarily left sided deficits in Finger Oscillation speed and Strength of Grip. Significant bilateral sensory deficits (suppressions) consistent with brain damage are also noted on the Sensory Perceptual Examination, with the left side being more impaired than the right (Chapter 4).

Pathognomonic Signs – As stated above, bilateral sensory suppressions were noted on the Sensory Perceptual Examination. There is also at least one questionable finding on the Aphasia Screening Test (on item 5, the patient responded, *"a star...or a rectangle...insignia...Nazis"*). Such a response can be considered an aphasic error and indicates a severe confusion and obvious loss of ability which is strongly suggestive of brain damage (4-51).

In summary, there are significant indications of brain impairment, including poor scores on the most sensitive indicators of cerebral dysfunction, severely lateralized deficits on motor and sensory examination, and a wide discrepancy between Verbal and Performance IQs on the WAIS. These findings support the contention that this individual's brain damage had resulted in significant cognitive and behavioral deficits.

2) What is the severity of brain damage?

Level of Performance – A Halstead Impairment Index of 1.0 suggests severe impairment. This level of severity is further confirmed by the profile sheet, which indicates that all scores are in the impaired range (2 or greater) and most approach the highest degree of dysfunction.

Pattern of Performance – An extreme difference between Verbal and Performance IQ scores (34 points), as well as the general depression of scores on the Halstead-Reitan Battery, strongly supports the hypothesis of severe impairment.

Right-Left Differences – Extreme differences between scores on the dominant and nondominant hands on Finger Oscillation and Strength of Grip suggest that the brain damage is severe.

Pathognomonic Signs – Sensory suppressions and the previously mentioned aphasic error are indications of clinically significant brain damage.

Almost all test scores suggest that the brain damage is severe and is contributing to significant deficits in problem-solving, motor and sensory abilities, and attention and concentration.

3) Is the lesion progressive or static?

Level of Performance – This patient's Performance IQ score is clearly inconsistent with his previous occupation, which is indicative of a decline. Both the Seashore Rhythm Test and Speech-sounds Perception Test are in the impaired range and had to be discontinued. Such poor overall performances would support a progressive, possibly tissue destructive lesion (Chapter 6).

Pattern of Performance – Since there is a significant difference between Verbal and Performance IQ, and the Seashore Rhythm and Speech-sounds Perception scores are both in the severely impaired range, a progressive lesion is suspected (Chapter 6).

Right-Left Differences – This method of inference yields little data with regard to this question.

Pathognomonic Signs – Significant sensory suppressions and one aphasic error add evidence to the progressive nature of this lesion.

In summary, this lesion appears to be of a progressive, space occupying nature.

4) Is the lesion diffuse or lateralized?

Level of Performance – This method of inference does not yield information which is pertinent to this question.

Pattern of Performance – The Performance IQ being 34 points lower than the Verbal IQ, even though usually considered a weak sign of lateralization, may be seen as a strong indication of right cerebral hemisphere involvement since there is such a significant difference (4-14). Seashore Rhythm, Speech-sounds Perception, and Trail Making A and B show no lateralizing relationships in this case since they were generally performed so poorly (Chapters 4 and 5).

Right-Left Differences – The Finger Oscillation Test and Strength of Grip Test both indicate significantly more impairment to the right cerebral hemisphere than to the left. This relationship is also demonstrated in the Sensory Perceptual Examination, where there are proportionately more errors on the left side of the body (Chapter 5). The TPT was performed so poorly that it does not add information when considering this question.

Pathognomonic Signs – Mild constructional dyspraxia on the Aphasia Screening Test, an aphasic error, and bilateral (but more strongly left sided) sensory suppressions on the Sensory Perceptual Examination present an inconsistent picture with regard to lateralization.

On the basis of left sided slowness and weakness on Finger Oscillation and Strength of Grip, an extremely low Performance IQ in relation to Verbal IQ, and more sensory deficits on the left side of the body, this lesion appears strongly lateralized to the right cerebral hemisphere, with some impairment of the left.

5) Is the impairment in the anterior or posterior part of the cerebral hemisphere?

Level of Performance – This method of inference does not yield useful information with regard to this question.

Pattern of Performance – Both Finger Oscillation and the Sensory Perceptual Examination are impaired, which suggests damage to the sensory and motor strip of the brain. Because of the generally poor performance on the TPT, no useful information for this question is added by this test. Anterior and posterior sections of the brain appear affected.

Right-Left Differences – This method of inference does not yield information regarding this question.

Pathognomonic Signs – Sensory suppressions and a very mild constructional dyspraxia implicate the posterior part of the cerebral hemispheres, but do not rule out anterior involvement.

This question is difficult to answer given these data; however, there are strong indications that both the sensory and motor strips are involved. Thus, the lesion is affecting the functioning of the anterior and posterior portions of the brain, particularly within the right cerebral hemisphere.

6) What is the most likely neuropathological process?

In review of the previous answers, this patient demonstrates severe, bilateral cerebral dysfunction with the right cerebral hemisphere being significantly more impaired than the left. The lesion is probably a progressive space occupying one which is exerting a significant effect on virtually all cognitive functions. The deficits are too lateralized to be associated with arteriosclerosis, degenerative disease, or infectious disorder, and the severity with partial sparing of verbal functions argues against both closed and penetrating head injuries. A CVA cannot be ruled out; however, one would expect more lateralized sensory deficits, fewer left sided motor abilities, and in the case of an old CVA, a better performance on tests such as TPT. This process of elimination leaves the results consistent with right intracerebral hemisphere neoplastic disease.

7) What are the implications for everyday functioning and treatment?

The prognosis associated with a glioblastoma is poor, and in this case, the chances of total remission are very low since this is the third time the patient has been operated on to remove the recurrent growth. The neuropsychological examination confirmed the serious effect that this lesion has had on the patient's ability to solve new problems, to think flexibly and efficiently, to exercise reasonable judgment, and to engage in tasks which require motor and sensory integrity. It was suggested that this individual be placed in a living situation which would be highly structured and supervised, with a focus on his reasonably intact verbal abilities.

References

Bach-Y-Rita, G., Lion, G. R., Climent, C. E., & Ervin, F. R. (1971). Episodic dyscontrol: A study of 130 violent patients. *American Journal of Psychiatry, 127*(11), 49-52.

Bailey, P. (1955). Symposium on the temporal lobe. *Archives of Neurology and Psychiatry, 74,* 568-569.

Bender, L. (1938). *A visual motor gestalt test and its clinical use.* New York: The American Orthopsychiatric Association.

Benton, A. L. (1963). *The Revised Visual Retention Test.* New York: Psychological Corporation.

Benton, A. L., Varney, N. R., & Hamsher, K. deS. (1978). Visuospatial judgment. *Archives of Neurology, 35,* 364-367.

Cameron, N. (1959). Paranoid conditions and paranoia. In S. Arieti (Ed.), *American handbook of psychiatry: Vol. 1.* New York: Basic Books.

Canter, A. (1970). *The Canter background interference procedure for the Bender-Gestalt Test: Manual for administration, scoring and interpretation.* Iowa City, Iowa: Iowa Psychopathic Hospital.

Christenson, A. L. (1975). *Luria's neuropsychological investigation.* New York: Spectrum.

Cullum, C. M., Steinman, D. R., & Bigler, E. D. (1984). Relationship between fluid and crystallized cognitive functions using Category Test and WAIS scores. *International Journal of Clinical Neuropsychology, VI, 3,* 172-174.

Daley, M. L., Swank, R. L., & Ellison, C. M. (1979). Flicker fusion thresholds in multiple sclerosis. *Archives of Neurology, 36,* 292-295.

Filskov, S. B., & Goldstein, S. G. (1974). Diagnostic validity of the Halstead-Reitan Neuropsychological Battery. *Journal of Consulting Psychology, 42,* 382-388.

Fishbach, R., Harrer, G., & Wagner, F. (1973). Veranderungen der flimmer-verschmelzungs frequenz bei multiple-sklerosekranken. *Meizinische Welt, 23,* 121-122.

Golden, C. J. (1978). *Diagnosis and rehabilitation in clinical neuropsychology,* Springfield, Ill.: Charles C. Thomas.

Golden, C. J. (1977). The validity of the Halstead-Reitan Battery in a mixed psychiatric and brain damaged population. *Journal of Consulting and Clinical Psychology, 45,* 1043-1051.

Goldstein, S. G., Daysack, R. E., & Kleinknecht, R. A. (1973). Effect of experience and amount of information on identification of cerebral impairment. *Journal of Consulting and Clinical Psychology, 41,* 30-34.

Gordon, R., Herman, G. T., & Johnson, S. A. (1975). Image reconstruction from projections. *Scientific American,* 56-68.

Graham, F. K., & Kendall, B. S. (1960). Memory for Designs Test: Revised general manual. *Perceptual and Motor Skills: Monograph supplement, 11,* 147-188.

Halstead, W. C. (1947). *Brain and intelligence.* Chicago: University of Chicago Press.

Heaton, R. K., & Crowley, T. J. (1981). Effects of psychiatric disorders and their somatic treatments on neuropsychological test results. In S. B. Filskov & T. J. Boll (Eds.), *Handbook of clinical neuropsychology.* New York: Wiley.

Heaton, R. K., & Pendleton, M. G. (1981). Use of neuropsychological tests to predict adult patients' functioning. *Journal of Consulting and Clinical Psychology, 49,* 807-821.

Hevern, V. W. (1980). Recent validity studies of the Halstead-Reitan approach to clinical neuropsychological assessment: A critical review. *Clinical Neuropsychology, 2,* 49-61.

Jarvis, P. E., & Barth, J. T. (1979). The neglect of physical-neurological factors in community mental health practice: A proposal for a better balance. *Clinical Neuropsychology, 3,* 20-23.

Jarvis, P. E., & Buchholz, D. J. (1981). Critical flicker fusion thresholds in subjects with multiple sclerosis. *Clinical Neuropsychology, 3,* 10-12.

Jarvis, P. E., & Vollman, R. R. (in press). Beyond the obvious: Two cases illustrating the need to consider both physical-neurological and psychosocial factors in assessment. *Clinical Neuropsychology.*

Klonoff, H., & Low, M. (1974). Disordered brain function in young children and early adolescents: Neuropsychological and electroencephalographic correlates. In R. M. Reitan & L. M. Davison (Eds.), *Clinical neuropsychology: Current status and applications.* Washington, D.C.: Winston.

Lezak, M. D. (1983). *Neuropsychological assessment* (2nd ed.). New York: Oxford University Press.

Luria, A. R. (1966). *Higher cortical functions in man.* New York: Basic Books.

Luria, A. R. (1973). *The working brain.* New York: Basic Books.

Matarazzo, J. D. (1972). *Wechsler's measurement and appraisal of adult intelligence* (5th ed.). Baltimore: Williams and Wilkins.

Messina (1977). Cranial computerized tomography: a radiologic-pathologic correlation. *Archives of Neurology, 34,* 602-607.

Meyer, V. (1961). Psychological effects of brain damage. In H. J. Eysenck (Ed.), *Handbook of abnormal psychology.* New York: Basic Books.

Parsons, O. A., & Miller, P. N. (1957). Flicker fusion thresholds in multiple sclerosis. *Archives of Neurology and Psychiatry, 77,* 134-139.

Reitan, R. M. (1955). Investigation of the validity of Halstead's measure of biological intelligence. *Archives of Neurology and Psychiatry, 73(28),* 28-35.

Reitan, R. M. (1959). *The effects of brain lesions on adaptive abilities in human beings.* Seattle: University of Washington.

Reitan, R. M. (1967). Psychological assessment of deficits associated with brain lesions in subjects with normal and subnormal intelligence. In J. L. Khanna (Ed.), *Brain damage and mental retardation: A psychological evaluation.* Springfield, Ill.: Charles C. Thomas.

Reitan, R. M. (1975). Assessment of brain-behavior relationships. In P. McReynolds (Ed.), *Advances in psychological assessment: Vol. 3.* San Francisco: Josey-Bass.

Reitan, R. M. (undated). *Manual for administration of neuropsychological test batteries for adults and children.* Seattle.

Reitan, R. M. (undated). *Neuropsychological methods of inferring brain damage in adults and children.* Unpublished.

Reitan, R. M., & Boll, T. J. (1971). Intellectual and cognitive functions in Parkinson's disease. *Journal of Consulting and Clinical Psychology, 37,* 364-369.

Reitan, R. M., & Davison, L. A. (1974). *Clinical neuropsychology: Current status and applications.* Washington, D. C.: Winston and Sons.

Reitan, R. M., & Tarshes, E. L. (1959). Differential effects of lateralized brain lesions on the Trail Making Test. *Journal of Nervous and Mental Disorders, 129,* 257.

Russell, E. W., (1975). A multiple scoring method for the assessment of complex memory functions. *Journal of Consulting and Clinical Psychology, 43*(6), 800-809.

Russell, E. W., Neuringer, C., & Goldstein, G. (1970). *Assessment of brain damage – A neuropsychological key approach.* New York: Wiley.

Shipley, W. C. (1946). *Institute of living scale.* Los Angeles: Western Psychological Services.

Starr, A., & Achor, L. J. (1975). Auditory brain stem responses in neurological disease. *Archives of Neurology, 32,* 761-768.

Steegmann, A. T. (1962). *Examination of the nervous system: A student's guide.* Chicago: Year Book Medical Publishers.

Swiercinsky, D. (1978). *Manual for the adult neuropsychological evaluation.* Springfield, Illinois: Charles C. Thomas.

Titcombe, A. F., & Willison, R. G. (1961). Flicker fusion in multiple sclerosis. *Journal of Neurology, Neurosurgery, and Psychiatry, 24,* 260-265.

Wechsler, D. (1945). A standardized memory scale for clinical use. *Journal of Psychology, 19,* 87-95.

Appendix

GLOSSARY

This glossary includes definitions of many of the technical terms used in this Guide as well as a number of other terms that the psychologist may encounter in both the neuropsychological and neurological literature and in reports of neurological examinations.

ABSENCE SEIZURES – Form of epilepsy in children characterized by a short altered state of consciousness (petit mal seizures).

ACALCULIA – Inability to perform simple mathematical calculations due to cerebral dysfunction.

ABSCESS – Circumscribed infection which is characterized by a build up of pus surrounded by a thick wall of cells.

AFFERENT FIBERS – Neuronal pathways which carry information upward toward the cerebral cortex from peripheral areas of the nervous system.

AGNOSIA – Inability to recognize sensory stimulation due to cerebral dysfunction.

AGRAPHIA – Inability to write due to cerebral dysfunction.

AKINESIA – Inability to move due to cerebral dysfunction.

ALEXIA – Inability to read due to cerebral dysfunction.

AMYGDALA – One of the structures of the limbic system which is located at the base of the temporal lobe.

ANEURYSM – The weak wall of a vein or artery which dilates and fills with blood. Such defective vascular areas may burst, causing hemorrhages of the adjacent tissue.

ANGIOGRAPHY – A radiological procedure to enhance pictures of the cerebral vasculature by taking x-rays of the head following the introduction of a radiopaque contrast material to a major artery.

ANGULAR GYRUS – A convolution of the cerebral cortex in the area of the parietal lobe which is intimately involved in the production of speech.

ANOMIA – Inability to name common items and figures due to cerebral dysfunction.

ANTERIOR COMMISSURE – Neuronal pathways which connect the temporal lobes.

ANTEROGRADE AMNESIA – Usually referred to as a loss of memory for events which follow cerebral trauma such as head injuries.

APHASIA – Inability to or deficit of communication due to cerebral dysfunction.

APRAXIA – Inability to initiate planned movements due to cerebral dysfunction.

ARACHNOID SPACE – One of the three layers of the meninges which is filled with fibrous tissue and acts as the conduit for cerebrospinal fluid to travel around the brain.

ARTERIOSCLEROSIS – Disease of the vascular system characterized by a build up of fatty deposits on the inner walls of veins and arteries, restricting blood flow throughout the brain.

ASTEREOGNOSIS – Inability to recognize simple and familiar objects and shapes due to cerebral dysfunction.

ASTROCYTOMA – Type of neoplasm which arises from astrocyte cells. These tumors are usually unencapsulated and intracerebral.

ATAXIA – Muscular incoordination associated with cerebral dysfunction.

ATROPHY – Shrinkage of (brain) tissue due to loss of neuronal processes.

AXON – The portion of a neuron which transmits energy from the cell body to the receptors of other neurons.

BASAL GANGLIA – Nuclei associated with the forebrain (amygdala, caudate nucleus, claustrum, globus pallidus, and putamen).

BILATERAL – Referring to both sides of the body or both cerebral hemispheres.

BITEMPORAL HEMIANOPSIA – Visual field loss in both temporal areas which is caused by damage to the optic chiasm.

BRAIN SCAN – Method of identifying neurological disturbances such as cerebrovascular accidents and neoplasms by injecting a radioisotope material into an artery and scanning the head with a Geiger counter to determine where the radioisotopes are collecting (in collections of blood, highly vascularized tumors, arteriovenus malformations, etc.).

BRAIN STEM – Thalamus, hypothalamus, basal ganglia, midbrain and hindbrain.

BROCA'S AREA (Aphasia) – A portion of the left frontal lobe located near the motor strip which is intimately involved in the production of speech. Disruption of this area can cause a Broca's aphasia which is characterized by deficits in expressive speech.

CENTRAL SULCUS (Fissure of Rolando) – A large fissure which separates the frontal and parietal lobes.

CEREBELLUM – A large structure which mediates motor coordination located in the posterior part of the brain below the occipital lobes.

CEREBROVASCULAR ACCIDENT – Ischemic disorder or disruption of blood flow in the brain due to an occlusion of a portion of the vascular system from a thrombus or embolus, or a hemorrhage.

CEREBROSPINAL FLUID (CSF) – A clear fluid produced by the choroid plexis in the ventricles and circulated around the brain and spinal cord through the subarachnoid space.

CINGULATE BODIES – Tissue found in the limbic system above the corpus callosum.

CONCUSSION – A head injury which is characterized by a loss of consciousness.

CONDUCTION APHASIA – An expressive aphasia which is characterized by an understanding of language, yet an inability to repeat words correctly.

CONSTRUCTIONAL DYSPRAXIA – Difficulty in reproducing (drawing) simple, geometric designs and objects.

CONTRECOUP – An effect in closed head injury which is characterized by damage to brain tissue at a location opposite the site of impact due to the brain's bouncing off the walls of the cranium.

CONTRALATERAL – Referring to the opposite side of the body or brain.

CONTRAST STUDY (X-ray) – Injection of a radiopaque dye into an artery, or air into the spinal column, followed by x-rays of the brain to highlight the cerebrovascular system or ventricle respectively.

CONTUSION – Injury to the vascular system which produces hemorrhaging and associated swelling.

CORPUS CALLOSUM – Intracerebral tissue connecting the right and left hemispheres.

CORTEX – The outer area or layer of brain tissue which is comprised of sulci and gyri.

CRANIAL NERVES – Twelve pairs of nerves which emanate from the brain and carry sensory and motor signals to and from the periphery of the central nervous system.

COMPUTERIZED AXIAL TOMOGRAPHY (CAT or CT Scan) – State of the art, computer assisted x-rays measuring densities of sections of the brain.

CYST – A sac of fluid usually associated with an infectious disorder.

DECEREBRATE (Rigidity) – Injury to the brain stem and/or cerebellum causing extension of limbs.

DEGENERATIVE DISEASE – Loss of neurons and cerebral atrophy, the most common of which is referred to as primary neuronal degeneration, or Alzheimer's disease.

DEMENTIA – Deterioration of mental functions characterized by cognitive decline and memory impairment.

DENDRITES – Receptor structures of a neuron which are characterized by branch-like projections.

DURA – The outermost layer of the meninges.

DYSARTHRIA – Difficulty in articulation.

DYSCALCULIA – Difficulty in performing simple arithmetic calculations.

DYSKINESIA – Difficulty in movement.

DYSLEXIA – Difficulty in reading.

DYSNOMIA – Difficulty in naming common objects and shapes.

DYSPHASIA – Difficulty in speech/communication.

EFFERENT FIBERS – Neuronal pathways which carry information downward from the cerebral cortex to the peripheral areas of the nervous system.

ELECTROENCEPHALOGRAPHY (EEG) – A method of recording bioelectrical discharge from the cortex of the brain through extradermal electrode placement.

ELECTROMYOGRAM (EMG) – A method of recording bioelectrical discharges from muscle groups.

EMBOLUS – An object such as an air bubble or blood clot which can become lodged in a vessel or artery causing an occlusion of blood flow.

ENCAPSULATED – An enclosure or covering, usually associated with the outer area of a neoplasm.

ENCEPHALITIS – Infection of the central nervous system.

ENCEPHALOMALACIA – Softening of brain tissue.

ENCEPHALOPATHY – Degeneration of the brain.

EPENDYMAL CELLS – Cells which comprise the inner layer of the ventricle walls.

EPILEPSY – Significant seizure disorder including classifications such as tonic-clonic, absence, and partial complex seizures.

EVOKED POTENTIALS – Measurement of the latency and wave form of visual and auditory signals.

EXTRACEREBRAL (Extrinsic) – Outside of the cerebral hemisphere, usually referring to neoplasms or cerebrovascular disruptions located between the skull and brain.

EXTRINSIC – See extracerebral.

FISSURE – Large sulcus or groove located in the cerebral cortex.

FRONTAL LOBES – The two largest areas of the brain anterior to the central sulcus (or Fissure of Rolando).

GERSTMANN SYNDROME – Disorder which is characterized by dyscalculia, dysgraphia, finger agnosia, and right-left confusion.

GLIAL CELLS – Connective tissue of the brain.

GLIOBLASTOMA (Multiforma) – Neoplasm arising from glial cells.

GLIOMA – See glioblastoma.

GRAY MATTER – Cells and connective tissue in the internal areas of the brain.

GYRUS (Gyri) – Convolutions which comprise the surface of the brain.

HEMATOMA – A build-up or pool of blood usually associated with the meninges of the brain.

HEMIPARESIS – Weakness affecting one side of the body.

HEMIPLEGIA – Paralysis affecting one side of the body.

HEMORRHAGE – Bleeding.

HIPPOCAMPUS – Anterior temporal lobe structure which is actively involved in memory function.

HOMONYMOUS HEMIANOPSIA – Loss of vision in one half of the visual field of both eyes (right temporal and left nasal, or right nasal and left temporal).

HYPOTHALAMUS – Structure dorsal to the thalamus which is involved in many behaviors such as sleeping, sexual activity, eating, and emotions.

IDEOKINETIC APRAXIA – Inability to carry out a motor activity without a reference object.

INFARCT – Dead (brain) tissue associated with an occlusion of the vasculature.

INTRACEREBRAL (Intrinsic) – Within the cerebral hemispheres, usually referring to neoplasms or cerebrovascular disruptions.

IPSILATERAL – The same side of the body.

ISCHEMIA – Lack of blood flow to an area of the brain or other organ.

INTRACRANIAL PRESSURE (ICP) – Level of pressure within the skull and cerebrospinal fluid system.

KORSAKOFF'S SYNDROME – Deterioration of the brain and cognitive abilities (particularly in memory) caused by chronic and severe alcohol abuse.

LACERATION – A tear or cut.

LATERAL FISSURE (Sylvian Fissure) – The deep sulcus or groove separating the temporal and parietal lobes.

LESION – Tissue damage.

LIMBIC SYSTEM – Interconnected structures in the brain (hippocampus, cingulate gyrus, septum, amygdala, olfactory bulb, mammillary bodies, and fornix) which are involved in emotional responses.

LUMBAR PUNCTURE – Insertion of a needle into the spinal column to remove cerebrospinal fluid for analysis and to determine level of intracranial pressure.

MEDULLA OBLONGATA – Structure of the brain below (and connected to) the pons and above the spinal cord.

MEDULLABLASTOMA – Neoplasm of the medulla oblongata.

MENINGES – Membranes which provide the venous drainage system of the brain, comprised of the dura mater, pia mater, and arachnoid.

MENINGIOMA – Neoplasm arising in the meninges.

MENINGITIS – Infection of the meninges.

METASTATIC NEOPLASM – Tumors which develop from abnormal cells which have migrated from another area of the body.

MOTOR NEURON – Neurons which emanate from the spinal cord and extend to muscles.

MYELIN SHEATH – Encompassing the axons of many nerves.

NEOPLASM – A tumor.

NEURON – A nerve cell in the brain which is comprised of a cell body, axon, and dendrites.

NEUROTRANSMITTER – A chemical substance which is released into the synaptic space between neurons to facilitate the chemical/electrical transmission of information between cells.

NUCLEAR MAGNETIC RESONANCE (NMR) – Computerized imagery based on the analysis of the magnetic properties of the substance of the brain and which resembles the pictures gathered from CAT scans.

OCCIPITAL LOBES – Posterior portion of the brain next to the parietal and temporal lobes.

OLIGODENDROGLIA – Glial cells which serve a support function in the brain.

OLIGODENDROGLIOMA – A neoplasm which arises from oligodendroglia.

OPTIC CHIASM – The area in which the optic nerves separate and cross over to the contralateral cerebral hemisphere. It is located in the basal portion of the brain, near the pituitary.

PAPILLEDEMA – Swelling of the optic disc due to increased intracranial pressure.

PARAPHASIA – Usually referred to as a communication deficit characterized by the substitution or addition of incorrect words into sentences.

PARIETAL LOBE – Portion of the brain which is posterior to the central sulcus and rostral to the temporal lobe.

PARKINSON'S DISEASE – A disorder which primarily involves the motor functions of the cerebellum and is characterized by tremors and gait deficits.

PERIPHERAL NERVES – Those nerves which lie outside of the central nervous system (brain and spinal cord).

PIA MATER – The portion of the meninges which lies directly above the brain.

PLASTICITY – Ability of the brain to compensate and change in response to brain injury.

PNEUMOENCEPHALOGRAPHY – Also referred to as "air studies" since it is characterized by the removal of some cerebrospinal fluid through a lumbar puncture and the replacement of that fluid with air. X-rays are then taken of the head after the air has traveled to the ventricles and through the arachnoid space. Such a procedure is designed to enhance the view of the ventricles and midline so that atropy, intracranial pressure, and the indirect results of neoplasms may be seen.

PONS – Large oblong structure in the area of the brain stem and comprised of motor fibers.

POSITRON EMISSION TOMOGRAPHY (PET Scan) – Sophisticated computer assisted x-ray procedure which is similar to the CAT scan and assesses the uptake and utilization of glucose within the brain.

POSTCENTRAL GYRUS – Convolution of the cerebral cortex which is located just posterior to the central sulcus and is involved in the mediation of sensory activity.

PRECENTRAL GYRUS – Convolution of the cerebral hemisphere which is located just anterior to the central sulcus and involved in the mediation of motor activity.

PTOSIS – A drooping eyelid associated with damage to the oculomotor cranial nerve.

RETICULAR ACTIVATING SYSTEM (Formation) – The portion of the brain stem which mediates level of systemic arousal.

ROENTGENOGRAPHY – X-ray photographic techniques.

SHEAR/STRAIN – The stretching or breaking of the axons and/or dendrites of nerves as a result of head trauma.

STEREOGNOSIS – The tactile recognition of objects and shapes.

STROKE – General classification for disorders of the brain which are characterized by a disruption of blood flow.

SULCUS – A groove or space between the gyri of the cerebral cortex.

SYNAPSE – The space between the terminal end of the axon and another cell body where neurotransmitters are released to carry signals from one nerve to another.

TEMPORAL LOBES – Areas of the brain located dorsal to the parietal lobes (separated from the parietal lobe by the lateral sulcus).

THALAMUS – Structures of the brain located to each side of the third ventricle and involved in some gross aspects of sensation.

THROMBUS – A blood clot which lodges in an artery or vessel, creating an occlusion.

TRANSIENT ISCHEMIC ATTACKS (TIA) – Having to do with short periods of insufficient blood supply to selected portions of the brain (usually involving small vasculature).

UNENCAPSULATED – See encapsulated.

UNILATERAL – Refers to one side of the body.

VENTRICLES – Four spaces within the brain through which cerebrospinal fluid circulates.

VESICLES (Synaptic) – Small structures at the terminal point of an axon, which contain the neurotransmitter substances.

VISUAL AGNOSIA – An inability to recognize common objects and shapes.

WERNICKE'S APHASIA – Inability to communicate verbally due to the impairment of receptive abilities.

WHITE MATTER – Connecting tissue within the brain.

XANTHROCHROMIA – Usually referred to as the discoloration of cerebrospinal fluid due to the presence of blood cells.

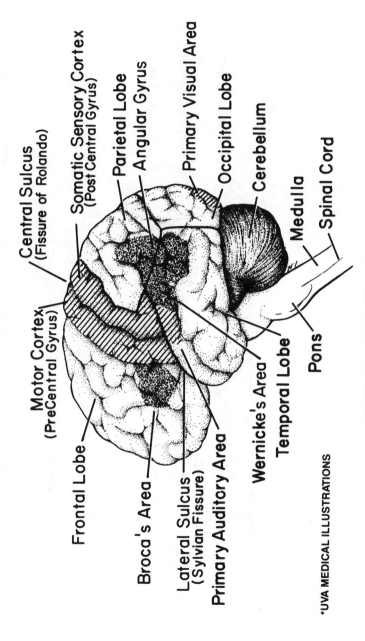

Central Sulcus
(Fissure of Rolando)

Somatic Sensory Cortex
(Post Central Gyrus)

Parietal Lobe

Angular Gyrus

Primary Visual Area

Occipital Lobe

Cerebellum

Medulla

Spinal Cord

Motor Cortex
(PreCentral Gyrus)

Frontal Lobe

Broca's Area

Lateral Sulcus
(Sylvian Fissure)

Primary Auditory Area

Wernicke's Area

Temporal Lobe

Pons

*UVA MEDICAL ILLUSTRATIONS

FIGURE A-1. LATERAL VIEW OF THE BRAIN

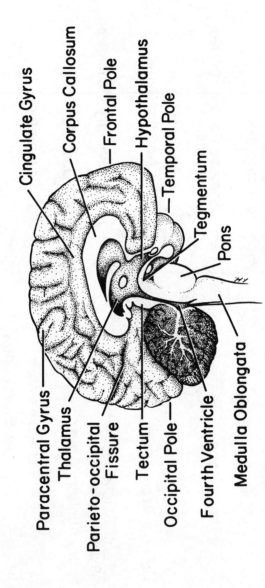

FIGURE A-2. MEDIAL VIEW OF INTERNAL STRUCTURES OF THE BRAIN

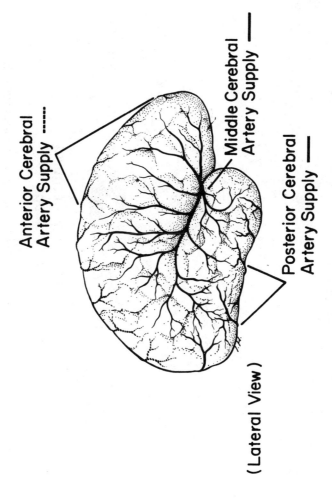

Anterior Cerebral
Artery Supply ----

Middle Cerebral
Artery Supply ——

Posterior Cerebral
Artery Supply ——

(Lateral View)

FIGURE A-3. LATERAL VIEW OF CEREBROVASCULAR SYSTEM

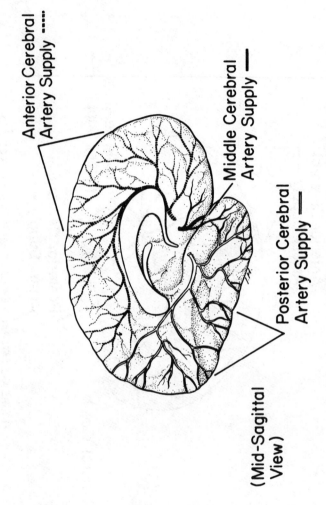

Anterior Cerebral Artery Supply ----

Middle Cerebral Artery Supply —

Posterior Cerebral Artery Supply —

(Mid-Sagittal View)

FIGURE A-4. MEDIAL VIEW OF CEREBROVASCULAR SYSTEM

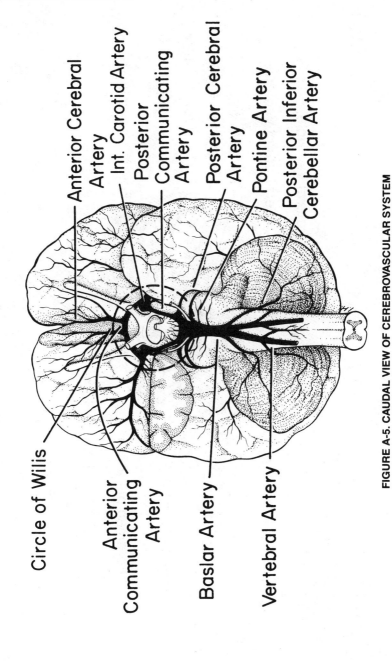

Anterior Cerebral Artery

Int. Carotid Artery

Posterior Communicating Artery

Posterior Cerebral Artery

Pontine Artery

Posterior Inferior Cerebellar Artery

Circle of Wilis

Anterior Communicating Artery

Baslar Artery

Vertebral Artery

FIGURE A-5. CAUDAL VIEW OF CEREBROVASCULAR SYSTEM

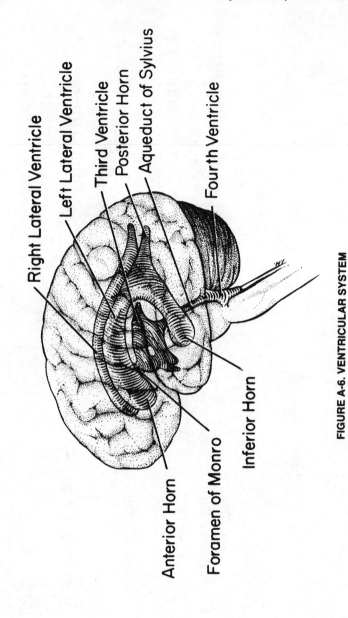

Right Lateral Ventricle

Left Lateral Ventricle

Third Ventricle

Posterior Horn

Aqueduct of Sylvius

Fourth Ventricle

Anterior Horn

Foramen of Monro

Inferior Horn

FIGURE A-6. VENTRICULAR SYSTEM

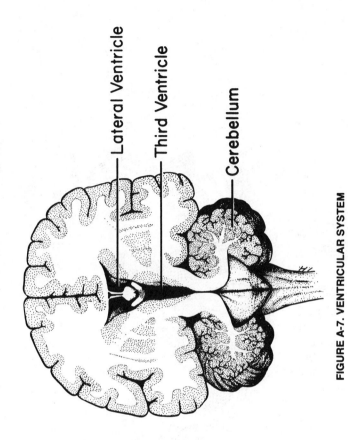

Lateral Ventricle

Third Ventricle

Cerebellum

FIGURE A-7. VENTRICULAR SYSTEM

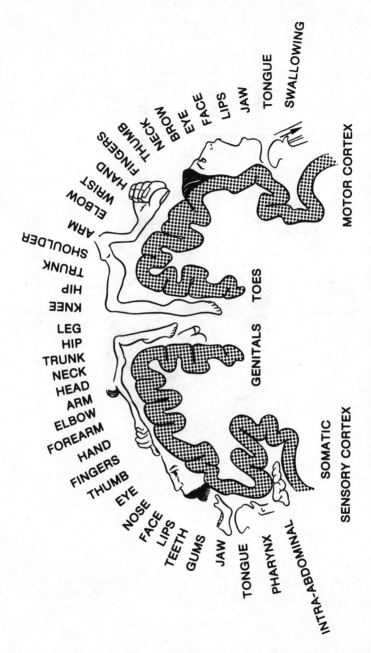

FIGURE A-8. FUNCTIONAL LOCATIONS ON SENSORY AND MOTOR STRIPS

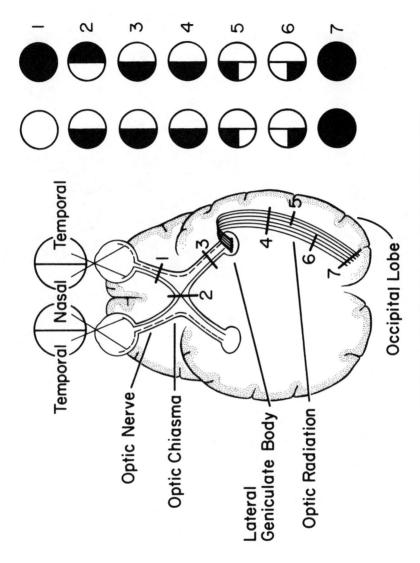

FIGURE A-9. OPTIC TRACTS AND VISUAL FIELD DEFICITS